Praise for *Yoga for Computer Users*

Sandy has a true gift for balancing technique with spirit, common sense with insight, modern application with traditional fundamentals. It is not often that computer users get a high-quality, inexpensive add-on with an upgrade path that can lead to enlightenment!

—Randy Nelson, Dean, Pixar University, Pixar Animation Studios

Yoga for Computer Users could change your life! Sandy Blaine deftly addresses the epidemic of problems that plague computer users and explains exactly what we can do about it. I have no doubt that anyone who reads this book will learn how to bring greater ease, comfort, and health into their life.

—Nora Isaacs, author of *Women in Overdrive: Find Balance and Overcome Burnout at Any Age*

This book is great preventive medicine for anyone who works at a computer. It's practical, clearly written, and full of good and simple advice on how to relax, release tense muscles, improve your posture, and bring yogic awareness into your work life.

—Timothy McCall, M.D., medical editor of *Yoga Journal*; author of *Yoga as Medicine: The Yogic Prescription for Health and Healing*

Yoga for Computer Users

Rodmell Press Yoga Shorts

By Sandy Blaine
Yoga for Computer Users
Yoga for Healthy Knees

By Shoosh Lettick Crotzer
Yoga for Fibromyalgia

By Judith Hanson Lasater, Ph.D., P.T.
Yoga Abs
Yoga for Pregnancy

rodmell press

YOGA SHOR

YOGA

FOR COMPUTER USERS

HEALTHY NECKS, SHOULDERS, WRISTS,
AND HANDS IN THE POSTMODERN AGE

▼　　▼　　▼　　▼　　▼　　▼　　▼　　▼　　▼

Sandy Blaine

RODMELL PRESS　　　BERKELEY, CALIFORNIA, 2008

Dedicated to my students, who are also my best teachers.

Library of Congress Cataloging-in-Publication Data

Blaine, Sandy.
 Yoga for computer users : healthy necks, shoulders, wrists, and hands
in the postmodern age / Sandy Blaine. — 1st ed.
     p. cm. — (Rodmell Press yoga shorts)
 Includes index.
 ISBN-13: 978-1-930485-19-8 (pbk. : alk. paper)
 ISBN-10: 1-930485-19-0 (pbk. : alk. paper)
 1. Hatha yoga—Therapeutic use. 2. Computer users—Health and hygiene.
 3. Overuse injuries—Prevention. I. Title.
 RM727.Y64B53 2008
 613.7'046—dc2   2007048590

Printed and bound in China
First Edition
ISBN-10: 1-930485-19-0
ISBN-13: 978-1-930485-19-8
12 11 10 09 08 1 2 3 4 5 6 7 8 9 10

Editor: Linda Cogozzo   Photographer: David Martinez
Associate Editor: Holly Hammond   Lithographer: Kwong Fat Offset Printing Co., Ltd.
Indexer: Ty Koontz   Text set in Dante
Cover and Text Design: Gopa & Ted2, Inc. Distributed by Publishers Group West

Contents

▼ ▼ ▼ ▼ ▼ ▼ ▼

Acknowledgments

▼ ▼ ▼ ▼ ▼ ▼ ▼ ▼ ▼ ▼ ▼

My heartfelt thanks go to everyone who supported me in writing this book.

My teacher and mentor Donald Moyer has been a source of inspiration, support, and opportunity for many years.

My publisher, Rodmell Press, has supported my work and made opportunity a reality in ways I had never dreamed of before working with them. This book is a collaborative effort made immeasurably better by Linda Cogozzo's skilled, precise, and respectful editing and the contribution of her ideas, which improved and expanded on my original concept. I am grateful, especially, for her supportive approach to the writing process as we worked together on this project.

I want to acknowledge my colleague Linda Burnham for her input and support. Linda's experience with healing her own RSI, and her willingness to share her journey in the great workshops she teaches, are a source of inspiration that I have drawn on here.

Friend and colleague Witold Fitz-Simon gave me support in various ways, including help with the Sanskrit terms used here.

I am grateful to my talented friend Joe Doebele, of TandemScientific.com, for his support and the generosity with which he shared his terrific editing and revising skills. He was an exceptional writing coach when I was under deadline pressure.

My longtime and always loving and generous friends, the Tricamo Palmer family (Regina, Blaine, Devlin, Julian, and Francesca), hosted me for a weeklong writing retreat so I could finish writing the book away from the pressures and distractions of work and home.

My friend and business partner, Betsy Weiss, was her usual stellar supportive self, and she held down the fort at the Alameda Yoga Station when I was busy writing.

I acknowledge all my yoga students for their continued support and appreciation of my work. I am grateful beyond words that so many dedicated yogis allow me to share my practice with them week after week, year after year.

Thank you to delightful teaching apprentice Connie Menzies for the breath-focused demo class that she taught as part of her training and for sharing her research and resources.

Inspiration and material for this book came particularly from my students at Pixar Animation Studios, where I taught my first ongoing classes over twelve years ago and continue to teach to this day. I would like to thank Pixar, especially the folks at Pixar University (Randy Nelson, Elyse Klaidman, Elizabeth Greenberg, and Adrienne Ranft), for sponsoring my classes there and supporting my work in a variety of ways.

Thank you to all the baristas at my favorite writing spots, where I spent countless hours with my laptop: Julie's Tea Garden, which is near my studio in Alameda, California, and where I've been known to spend days on end writing, researching, and sipping organic chai lattes out on the garden patio; the fantastic bakery/café Sweet Adeline in Oakland, and Crema, my favorite office-away-from home in Portland, Oregon.

It was in writing this book that I discovered firsthand how truly useful yoga can be in counteracting the detrimental effects of computer use.

In autumn 2006, nearing the end of this book and facing an impending editorial deadline, I took a week off from teaching yoga and went out of town on a self-imposed writing retreat. I went to Portland, Oregon, where I have friends and family and which is something of a home way from home for me. There I was largely away from the distractions and demands of my yoga studio, my telephone, and all the undone projects and errands that needed attending to at home.

For that one week, I lived the life of a writer. For the first time in many years, I structured my day not around my yoga practice but instead spent each morning with my laptop at a café. In many ways, this week of focusing on writing was a great luxury, but it was also, quite instructively, a window into another way of life, and for better and worse I got to experience directly what it is like to be desk- and computer-bound.

Although I did not ever write for more than four hours at a stretch, and I took a long walk or attended a yoga class every afternoon after writing, it was remarkable how different my body felt when I regularly started the day at the computer. Accustomed to feeling vital and relaxed and continually renewed from my daily practice, I was hyperaware of how tight my muscles felt and how much more constricted my breath was following even just one medium-length computer session. My body craved yoga simply for maintenance. The physical and mental effects of continual computer use are cumulative, and they may be hard to discern as they creep up on a person over months or years. For me, having a different experience to compare it to, it was easy to see how much I needed to take my own advice!

It is from this newly discovered perspective that I offer the guidelines I've put forth here for taking care of ourselves in the technological age. Yoga, practiced with dedication and mindfulness, offers this remarkable opportunity: To feel good in our bodies as we move about in the world. When the demands of our daily lives lead us in the direction of physical discomfort, injury, and premature aging, it is all the more important that we use whatever resources are available to us to counteract those stresses. With yoga, we can perhaps slow down the aging process a bit and stay strong, supple, and balanced for longer, so we can more fully enjoy our existence. I hope that the program in this book will give you some tools to bring greater ease into your life.

Part One

Moving Forward: The Human Body in the Technological Age

▼　▼　▼　▼　▼　▼　▼　▼　▼　▼　▼

Necessary Steps and Changes

THE HUMAN BODY evolved to hunt and gather, to run and jump and climb, to play hard and rest fully—not to sit in front of a computer all day. Evolution has not kept up with the rapid changes of the technological age; we are simply not equipped to deal with all the requirements of modern life. Many of us need or choose to spend most of our days working at a computer. But this lifestyle takes its toll, sometimes a heavy one, in a variety of specific ways, including spine and back problems; shoulder, neck, and upper back tension; and a variety of repetitive stress injuries, such as carpal tunnel syndrome and tendonitis. As if that weren't enough, one of the most significant physiological effects of stress is a weakened immune system, which impairs the body's natural ability to prevent or recover from such injuries. It is likely that each major change in the way people live has brought with it an evolutionary challenge to the human body, and history proves there is no going back. Instead we must find solutions and continue to evolve. With this book, I hope to offer some yoga-based remedies to all these problems. To start with, it is important to understand a bit about the anatomical and physiological effects of prolonged computer use.

First, if you spend most of your day at a computer, you are at risk for repetitive stress injury (RSI). Even using a phone or personal data assistant (PDA) to send text messages can cause certain conditions that relate to the nerves of the hands when they are overused. Many other activities can cause RSI; for example, musicians, seamstresses, and chefs all regularly seek treatment, and what they have in common is the demand that their work places on their arms and hands. Until the computer age, however, RSI never approached the epidemic proportions we see now.

Second, whether or not you currently have symptoms, knowing that you're at risk makes implementing some kind of preventative self-care regimen well worth considering. It's like having a genetic predisposition to a certain disease: the people I know who are prone toward hypertension eat a low-sodium diet and exercise regularly to reduce the stresses on their bodies that might lead to more serious problems. For computer users, a proactive preventative regimen can help keep problems from developing. Although it may be contrary to human nature to treat a problem that doesn't yet exist, prevention is always more effective than any cure. This is especially so in the case of RSI, because nerve damage often reaches the stage where it is irreversible. I've seen people lose the use of their hands to the point where they can't drive a car, turn a doorknob, or hold a teacup.

Finally, although the program of yoga exercises suggested in this book can do much to help you prevent RSI and may even ease minor symptoms, it will be effective only if followed regularly. If you are working (or playing) at the computer eight hours a day or more, an occasional half hour of yoga is not likely to be enough to counteract the demands those hours of repetitive muscle use and nerve signals are putting on your body and mind. Pausing for regular stretching breaks whenever you are at the computer is great for starting to counteract the effects of prolonged computer use, and consistency is key to realizing continued benefits rather than just momentary relief. For even better results, those long hours of repetitive movement should be balanced with a full exercise program, including a complete yoga practice. Toward that end, later in this book you'll find suggestions and sequences for focused yoga practice away from the computer. Ideally these would be sessions lasting thirty to forty-five minutes, in the morning or at the end of the day, or both.

It is important to note that acute RSI is a medical condition that requires medical supervision. The program outlined in this book focuses on prevention; it does not offer a cure for advanced RSI. The same exercises that can help keep muscles and nerves healthy are not necessarily recommended for nerves that are already significantly damaged; these generally require very different treatment. In severe cases of RSI, the nerves may be beyond repair and may need therapies to minimize and manage pain. If you do have RSI symptoms that indicate nerve damage—that is, if you are experiencing chronic pain or weakness in certain areas—you should consult a doctor before beginning any treatment.

Even with serious, debilitating RSI, although managing the disease may require major lifestyle changes, you can probably find ways of relieving your symptoms, at least to some extent. Although the best treatment varies from person to person, a variety of activities and therapies in addition to yoga have been helpful to RSI patients. These include swimming, t'ai chi and qigong, dance, massage therapy, acupuncture, chiropractic treatment, or some combination of these. Even when you find a program that manages your symptoms effectively, the damaged areas will most likely always be vulnerable, so you must make space in your life to consistently follow a self-care program to keep getting the benefits. And if you don't want your hands, wrists, and shoulders to deteriorate to the point of dysfunction, you also must find ways to change the things you're doing that are causing and/or aggravating your symptoms.

The thought that we must make radical changes in our lifestyles, work habits, or even our careers to protect our health can be daunting. But our computerized society is facing a serious epidemic that must be dealt with. Ergonomics, exercise, and massage may help, and while other therapies and even cures for RSI may be on the way, for the moment, taking care of yourself by removing the cause is, by far, the most effective self-care option if you are in severe pain. Again, not letting it get to that point is clearly preferable. This means that, as soon as you experience any initial symptoms, taking immediate steps to change how, or how much, you work at your computer and devoting as much time as possible to balancing computer use with a preventative exercise and relaxation regimen. If it seems impossible to slow down, think about the outcome if you don't. Once RSI has set in to the point that you can't use the computer without pain, it may very well be too late. Rarely can any treatment effectively repair that level of nerve damage, so the decision to change careers will have been made for you.

How Yoga Can Help

I believe wholeheartedly in yoga as a highly effective and beneficial healing modality for preventative self-care. I have practiced yoga for twenty years and have used it to heal a variety of my own medical conditions (most notably, rehabilitating my badly injured knees). Moreover yoga has helped my students and a number of close friends cope with RSI and other computer-related health challenges.

Although here we focus primarily (though not solely) on the upper body, a full yoga program uses virtually all of the body's voluntary muscles. No other discipline that I'm aware of can make this claim, and the great majority of them require some type of repetitive movement that, in spite of the benefits it may offer, also eventually causes problems. The health benefits to using the entire musculoskeletal system are numerous. In particular, the increased range of motion and circulation yoga brings to the body is especially helpful in combating RSI and in providing countermovements to the habitual, damaging, "computer slump" posture, which causes your muscles to lock up and your back to suffer. Yoga is an antidote to the stagnation of energy that occurs in your body as you sit at your computer hour after hour.

In addition to the essential musculoskeletal benefits, yoga also offers a unique stress management system, alternating between physical exertion and deep relaxation, which trains the nervous system to turn off the stress response. We will discuss the practical application of relaxation and meditation to health management in more detail, as we look at the detrimental physiological effects of stress and how best to avoid them.

A Healthy Musculoskeletal System

Muscles suffer, albeit in different ways, from both overuse and underuse. A muscle that is constantly contracting and is never stretched becomes hard and tight, restricting movement; these tight muscles can literally pinch the associated nerves, leading to painful sensation. Muscles that are rarely accessed become slack and can feel dull and inert; under or unused nerve pathways weaken the mind-body connection, and there can be loss of sensation.

Muscles stay youthful, supple, and healthy when they are regularly both contracted and stretched. Anytime you stretch a muscle, the opposing muscles contract to create and maintain the stretching action, so yoga poses create both flexibility and strength in a related group of muscles. For example, when you bend your elbow and flex your biceps, your triceps muscles, on the opposite side of the upper arm, must stretch to create that action, and vice versa—the biceps must contract in order to stretch out the triceps. Muscles continue to work in complementary opposition to hold you in position for as long as you continue in a stretch. Thus yoga employs a healthy, purifying "squeeze and soak" action, as the muscles respond to this alternating contraction and extension by releasing toxins, much like a wet washcloth releases moisture when it is wrung out. When the muscles relax again after being used, fresh supplies of blood and oxygen flow in.

Muscles that are equally supple and strong translate to joints that are both mobile and supported, creating a structurally sound body and the ease of movement and energy flow that we associate with youth. In fact, it is possible to retain or restore suppleness, develop greater strength, and keep your entire musculoskeletal system youthful far later in life if you take care of yourself wisely.

Chairs and the Human Back

The spinal column is arguably the most important single part of the body. The spine provides the body's main structural support, including, for humans, the ability to both stand and sit upright. It is the conduit for messages to flow back and forth between the body and the brain. The spine has always been vulnerable to injury and back problems, especially of the lower back, are an extremely common complaint. Whether or not you suffer from back problems, you probably know people who do. Some studies estimate that up to 70 percent of people over forty have back problems. If that's true, something is clearly wrong.

Chairs, and the amount of time we spend sitting in them, are major culprits. Put a computer or a steering wheel in front of us, and the strain on our posture is compounded. Tight hip and leg muscles (which are more common than not in adults who don't stretch and are further tightened by a life spent sitting in chairs) add even more stress, because they reduce the mobility of the hip sockets, in effect "gluing" the pelvis to the thighbones and limiting the ability of the hip joints to contribute to healthy posture in the way that nature intended. As ball-and-socket joints, the hips should ideally support the spine by rolling easily up and over the thighbones to help you sit up all the way from the sacrum (the base of the spine). When this movement is restricted, the smaller and much more vulnerable sacroiliac and lumbar vertebral joints are forced to take over and try to do a job they're not made for. The result is that untold numbers of back injuries occur, as these joints and the related muscles strain to support our seated posture, pulling against gravity and our own tight muscles.

This condition inevitably leads to poor posture, which in turn causes or at least contributes to neck and shoulder tension. Holding the body in relatively still or uncomfortable positions for long periods, or just unconsciously holding tension in the muscles (tensing certain muscles when we are feeling stressed or simply out of habit), instill unhealthy patterns in those muscles, eventually resulting in problems like chronic pain, tension headaches, and other maladies.

RSI: What and Why

Historically the knees and the spine have always been the most injury-prone areas of the body. Only in the age of computers has the vulnerability of the arms and hands been fully revealed. Having taught yoga classes and RSI prevention seminars for high-tech companies over the past dozen years, I have seen firsthand, again and again, how damaging the combination of stress and the physical requirements of continual computer use can be. This damage is known medically as repetitive stress injury, which describes a myriad of physical complaints, from severe neck and shoulder tension to tendonitis to carpal tunnel syndrome.

While neither the cause nor the cure for RSI is well understood, it does seem that computer workers are particularly vulnerable to RSI-type problems, probably due to a combination of long hours of sitting in a chair hunched over a keyboard, the repetitive movement of both the small and large muscles of the upper body that is required for using a keyboard and mouse, and pressures such as work deadlines that keep the nervous system in overdrive.

People are often puzzled about how neck and shoulder tension can cause pain in the hands and wrists. It has to do with a series of related nerve pathways, but in the big picture it is always the smaller joints and muscles that suffer when the larger ones aren't able to do their jobs effectively. For example, when someone has tight hamstrings, it is often the lower back that sustains the damage, as the much smaller and more vulnerable lumbar and sacroiliac joints try to compensate for reduced mobility in the hip joints. Overly tight hip rotators are similarly most often experienced as knee pain and even injuries, because they impede healthy movement of the legs. Likewise when the neck, shoulder, and upper back muscles are constricted, the small muscles and joints of the wrists and hands, which are already working harder at the keyboard than nature intended, are adversely affected by lack of mobility in the larger ones.

The Physiological Effects of Stress

Although stress may begin in the brain, it is not just a mental concept or state of mind. Rather it is a normal, in fact inevitable, reaction to stimuli, whether internal or external, real or imagined, which produces a whole slew of physiological reactions in the body.

We know that stress affects the musculoskeletal system. How often have you become aware, after hours of working at the computer, that your shoulders have been creeping up around your ears, the muscles of your upper back and neck are becoming tighter and tighter, and, if you are under pressure, you are clenching your belly? Most often stretching and breathing—the fundamentals of yoga—will do a great deal to alleviate the muscular symptoms of stress.

Less obvious is how stress affects the body's internal systems, including the nervous system and the regulation of its delicate and complex hormonal balance. And while the body is built to withstand a certain amount of stress, in modern life our nervous systems are often in overdrive, and our bodies are oversaturated with stress hormones, due to constant tension. For a clear and entertaining medical explanation of exactly how chronic stress affects the different systems of the body, I recommend the work of Robert M. Sapolsky, particularly his book *Why Zebras Don't Get Ulcers*, which covers stress physiology and stress-related disease in detail. Here suffice it to say that the human body developed to cope with short-term stress, particularly physical crises, and not the kinds of chronic stressors we face in modern life.

When there is too much ongoing stress, the body spends most of its energy responding to it and doesn't have enough left for repair and maintenance, so physical systems like digestion, reproduction, and, perhaps most significantly, the immune system are not able to function optimally. Because of this, an over-stressed body is less able to deal with the wear and tear on the muscles, joints, and nerves caused by long hours at the computer. Along with the damage the body sustains, the natural healing process is simultaneously impaired.

This reality makes the relaxation component of yoga an essential part of any preventative self-care or healing program designed to deal with RSI and other detrimental effects of computer use. Regular, deep relaxation tones the nervous system, and the body functions at its best when it is well rested. So the relaxation exercises at the end of a yoga practice are not just a "reward" for having exercised; they are an integral component of caring for your health and well-being in general and your immune system in particular.

How to Use This Book

The rest of this book outlines a yoga-based self-care program designed to deal with the challenges to our health that a computer-centered lifestyle presents. The program is made up of several complementary elements.

The section that follows gives suggestions for balancing your computer time with healthy self-care breaks, guidelines to keep in mind as you begin taking yoga breaks, including some ideas to help you practice in a work environment, and, most important, instructions for specific, beneficial yoga exercises—*asanas* (yoga poses and stretches), *pranayama* (yogic breathing techniques), and meditation practices. The focus of the exercises chosen for this section is on developing the components of a healthy seated posture and on improving the tone, suppleness, and circulation in the muscles of the upper body, thus creating both more mobility and increased awareness of healthy movement in the joints. Along with the instructions for performing the exercises are descriptions of the particular benefits of each one and some cautions to keep in mind. Yoga practice requires a minimal amount of equipment, and each pose includes an explanation of the props you will need and how to use them.

Most of the exercises in this first section can be practiced while at your computer or when taking a short break from it. For maximum benefit, I recommend doing these stretches regularly throughout your time at the computer and, for those working regular business hours, taking at least two focused, 10-to-20-minute yoga breaks during the course of a full workday. Before jumping in, however, keep in mind that reading the whole book, especially the practice guidelines, before you begin practicing the exercises will help ensure that you get the best results from your yoga practice.

Part 3 outlines how to approach a focused (computer-free) yoga practice, perhaps before or after work. This section adds a few more asanas, which are intended to help you get the most out of your personal yoga practice in terms of balancing your body (especially the musculoskeletal and nervous systems) with the particular stresses of prolonged computer use. Each exercise includes full instructions, an explanation of the benefits, required and suggested equipment, and some cautions to keep in mind. Whether your computer time is regular or sporadic, starting and ending each day with twenty to thirty minutes of yoga is a wonderful and effective antidote to the demands that heavy computer use places on the body, mind, and spirit.

Part 4 gives several suggested practice sequences that you can use to guide your yoga practice, depending on how much time you have and what your particular needs are at the time. This section also covers the basic guidelines and requirements for a safe and effective yoga practice. For the best results, alternate the different sequences, and keep the practice guidelines in mind.

Part 5 includes some ideas and suggestions for incorporating yoga into your everyday life as well as some resources for further developing your practice. I hope these will be helpful as you begin to care for yourself more fully and enjoy the benefits of a healthier, freer, more joyful experience of working with and living in your body.

Part Two

Desktop Yoga

▼ ▼ ▼ ▼ ▼ ▼ ▼ ▼ ▼ ▼ ▼

Take a Break! Balancing Yoga Practice with Computer Time

WHETHER YOU ARE using the computer for work, play, or some combination, the more hours you spend on it, the more you need to balance those hours with time devoted to taking care of yourself. This is the essential concept of counterbalance. When I teach an introduction to yoga class, one question I am often asked is whether one yoga class a week is enough. There is no simple answer to that. First of all, it begs the question, enough for what? One class a week is certainly and infinitely better than no yoga at all, and probably it is enough to begin noticing some improvement in physical well-being, especially in the hours directly following the class. The benefits begin to dissipate as time goes on, however, and once a week is definitely not enough to compensate for forty hours a week or more spent at the computer, any more than one meal that includes vegetables is enough to counterbalance twenty previous meals of sugar and fat. More consistent practice reaps more ongoing benefits, because when you practice multiple times per week, there is less time for your muscles to tighten and for stresses to accumulate between practices. Thus, as you add more yoga to your weekly or even daily life, the benefits become both cumulative and exponential.

The first step in alleviating the physical and mental stresses of computer activity is to pause for periods of regular stretching and breathing, breaking up the time you spend using your keyboard and mouse by alternating it with time spent doing countermovements, and focusing inward instead of on your screen. The exercises that follow can be done throughout the day to help alleviate those stresses. While some of them may be more comfortable for practice in private than in a communal working environment, all of them can be practiced easily in a small space, many of them while sitting at your desk. Before we get to the exercises themselves, a few words about practicing yoga at work are in order for those whose computer use is primarily on the job.

Practicing at Work: Issues and Suggestions

Although there was a time when yoga was considered a quirky, counterculture pursuit, or even just plain weird, in the past decade it has entered the mainstream exercise world. Most people today think of yoga just as they do any other health practice or form of exercise. Hopefully your colleagues will support you in taking care of your health and be as accepting of a yoga break as they would be of a run or a tennis game at lunchtime. Every workplace is different, however. You will have to gauge how much acceptance and support you will get at yours and set up your practice space and schedule accordingly. In any case, the workplace obviously does not offer the same kind of privacy that you get practicing at home.

If you have a private office, perhaps you can just shut the door to close off your space for practice. If your office has windows, curtains or some other window covering may be needed so you can practice unselfconsciously. If you have a large enough office, maybe you can dedicate a corner of it to be your personal yoga space. But even if you have just enough room to lay down your mat, you have enough space to do a reasonably complete yoga practice. Taking a few moments to set up your mat and props and to put your computer in sleep mode will help create a bubble of space around you to separate yourself from work and move fully into practice. Decide ahead of time how long you want your practice session to be, and try not to answer calls or check e-mail for the duration.

Working in a cubicle or open floor plan is a different matter entirely, as your space and privacy will be so much more constrained. If you can't find a quiet, private space, such as an empty conference room, in which to practice, you may want to limit yourself to only the seated exercises for your office yoga breaks and save the ones that require more freedom for home, or at least for times when you are alone in the office. Another option, though, is organizing a community practice with your workmates. You may find that it stirs up interest when you begin to practice at work. Consider offering to teach your colleagues these exercises or even to lead a group practice on a regular basis. More people participating will solve the problem of self-consciousness, and it can also be very motivating.

The Poses: Take a Break from Your Computer

Seated Posture

▼ ▼ ▼ ▼ ▼ ▼ ▼ CREATES AWARENESS AND
SUPPORT FOR A HEALTHY SPINE

CAUTIONS: Use a lift under the sitting bones if you have
lower back problems or very tight hips or hamstrings.

PROP: 1 chair

OPTIONAL: 1 wedge or 1 nonskid mat or 1 blanket • 2nd nonskid mat

This first exercise, which covers the basics of healthy posture and learning how to (and how not to) sit in your chair, is essential in itself. It also sets up the basic starting position for many of the following exercises. Many of these exercises are done seated, so it is essential to start with an exercise-friendly chair. Yoga classes often use basic metal folding chairs, and these are ideal because they are stable and provide a firm surface. If you don't have one of these available, other chairs can work, but the more basic, the better. Note that the chair you use for your yoga practice has different requirements than the best ergonomic choice for your computer workstation (for more information on this issue, see the section on props, in Part 4). For our purposes, using a chair with wheels is not safe, and arms will get in the way of many movements.

For those with tight hamstrings or hips, using a lift under the sitting bones is an important modification for supporting a healthy back and good posture. The same prop can also help compensate for weakness of the core abdominal and lower back muscles or adjust for your proportions (for example, your height relative to the size of the chair). The ideal chair height allows your knees to be at the same height as your hip sockets or slightly lower. If you are tall, when you sit in the chair and place your feet flat on the floor your knees may be pushed up higher than your hip sockets. This is not a good position for your back in this stretch (or in general, in fact), so in this case you definitely want to use a prop under your sitting bones so your thighs can drop a bit lower than the pelvis. There is no downside, only benefit, to taking advantage of this option. A hard foam wedge, a folded nonskid mat, or a firm blanket (folded several times) are all good props for lifting the pelvis, and you can experiment with these to create the most comfortable and stable seated position for yourself (Figure 1A). Even if you don't need a lift under your sitting bones to support your posture,

FIGURE 1A
SEATED POSTURE, WITH SUPPORT

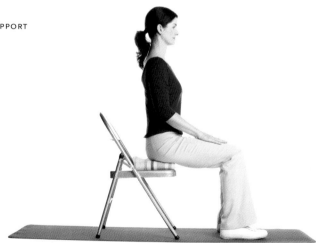

a nonskid mat folded over the seat of the chair can make the seated poses more comfortable; the seat of a metal folding chair can be slippery, cold, or just plain uncomfortable because the surface is so hard. If the floor is slippery, place a second nonskid mat under it for stability. If you are practicing barefoot and the floor surface is uncomfortable (as might be an industrial carpet in an office), this mat on the floor can also provide a more comfortable pad for your feet.

Sit at the very edge of the chair seat, with your feet hip-width apart and firmly planted on the mat. If you are using a prop to lift your sitting bones, it should also go at the edge of the chair seat. Move your weight forward so you are sitting toward the front edge of your sitting bones, rather than rolling back onto your gluteal muscles (the large muscles of the buttocks). Ideally you want to feel these bones pressing slightly into the chair or your prop.

Place your hands on your hips, and let your pelvis rock slightly up and down so the muscles of the hip sockets loosen up and you find the most upright position for the pelvis. The front hipbones should be lifting slightly off the thighbones, and the sacrum should be moving in and up toward your head, rather than slumping back toward the back of the chair. This rocking motion of the pelvis should help you feel the healthy movement of the hip sockets rolling over the thighbones and also the difference between a collapsed spine and a spine that is supported by the rotation and lift of the pelvis.

Once you have found this upright position, maintain it as you place your hands on your thighs and relax your shoulders (Figure 1B). Close your eyes to help with focus, and become more aware of your alignment. Ideally you want to feel the shoulders balanced directly above the pelvis and the crown of the head placed as precisely as possible over the tailbone. To create healthy posture, rather than pulling up with the back muscles, continue to lift from the hip sockets and sacrum, and lengthen up through the crown of the head, keeping the back of the neck and skull long, and the chin relaxed, with the jaw parallel to the floor. As you create more length between the tailbone and the crown of the head, feel a sense of space opening up between the vertebrae, and let the head feel as light as possible, like a helium-filled balloon floating up from a string. The string is your spine, anchored to the chair by your tailbone.

Try to hold Seated Posture for at least 1 minute, and when that is comfortable, gradually work up to a longer hold time. You can use this exercise to begin your in-office yoga practice, and it should also be practiced at regular intervals throughout the day. In reality, you are going to slump sometimes. The human body was not meant to sit for hours on end, so be gentle with yourself when you catch your spine collapsing, and come back to this exercise. If you practice it regularly, while you won't always have perfect posture, your posture will continually improve, and you will find that your body self-corrects more easily, and eventually automatically, as it learns to support and even prefer a healthier position.

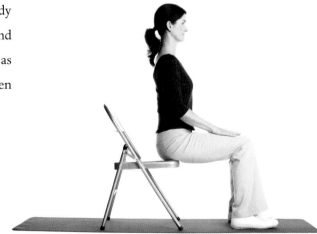

FIGURE 1B
SEATED POSTURE

Seated Mountain Pose with Basic Arm Stretch

PARVOTASANA

▼ ▼ ▼ ▼ ▼ ▼ ▼ OPENS THE SHOULDER JOINTS • RELEASES
SHOULDER TENSION • LENGTHENS THE INTERCOSTAL MUSCLES

CAUTION: Practice with care in the case of shoulder injuries.

PROP: 1 chair

OPTIONAL: 1 wedge or 1 blanket or 1 nonskid mat • 2nd nonskid mat • 1 block

Begin in Seated Posture (Figure 1A or Figure 1B). Clasp your hands with your fingers interwoven, so when you turn your palms away from you, the fingers are against the backs of the hands. Place your clasped hands on top of your head, with your palms turned upward and your fingers touching your head. Lengthen your spine by gently pressing the crown of your head into your hands. Next, straighten your arms, keeping your fingers interlaced and stretching your palms upward, as if you could place them on the ceiling (Figure 2A). Try not to let your arms

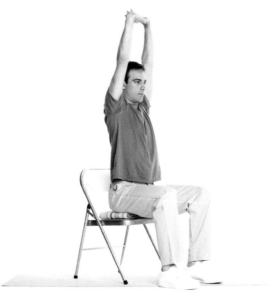

FIGURE 2A
SEATED MOUNTAIN POSE WITH BASIC ARM STRETCH

come forward, but rather stretch them straight up, so that the biceps are along-side your ears.

As the arms stretch upward and toward each other, try to keep the tops of the shoulders soft and the shoulder blades wide, so the inner upper shoulder muscles don't become overly hard or squeezed. Moving the arms up and in while keeping the shoulder blades wide are two opposing actions, so you'll need to play one against the other to find the stretch that feels best to you. You should feel the stretch primarily along the sides of the torso, all the way through the side chest and armpits, and even into the triceps muscles of the upper arms. You may also feel a gentle stretch of the hands and wrists, which is fine, but don't overdo this. The focus of the stretch, and the main sensation, should be at the outer shoulder joints.

If it is difficult to clasp the hands or to straighten the arms in this position, an option is to hold a block between the palms instead. In this version, the palms are flat along the sides of the blocks, and pressing the roots of the fingers and the thumb pads (the part of the palm between the thumb and index finger and at the base of the thumb) into the block as you stretch your arms overhead, reaching your fingertips upward toward the ceiling (Figure 2B).

Relax and breathe in this stretch for approximately 1 minute, and then release and repeat one more time, with the hands interlaced the opposite way. You can achieve this opposite handclasp by moving each finger over one position, so the opposite index finger becomes the one closer to the thumbs.

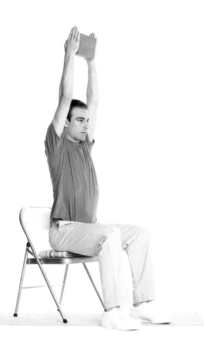

FIGURE 2B
SEATED MOUNTAIN POSE WITH
BASIC ARM STRETCH, WITH BLOCK

Reverse Prayer Pose

PASCHIMA NAMASKAR

▼ ▼ ▼ ▼ ▼ ▼ ▼ OPENS THE SHOULDER JOINTS AND CHEST •
RELEASES SHOULDER AND NECK TENSION • STRETCHES
THE HANDS AND WRISTS • FREES THE BREATH

CAUTIONS: Practice with care in the case of shoulder, hand, or wrist injuries.

PROP: 1 chair

OPTIONAL: 1 wedge or 1 blanket or 1 nonskid mat • 2nd nonskid mat

Begin in Seated Posture (Figure 1A or Figure 1B). Lengthen your spine and stretch your arms out to your sides in a T position. Moving from inside the shoulder sockets, begin to internally rotate both arms until the palms of the hands turn as far back as possible. When the arms have rotated as far as is comfortable, bend the elbows, bringing the hands behind the back with the middle fingers touching, the little fingers pressing gently against the back, and the palms facing downward toward the seat of the chair.

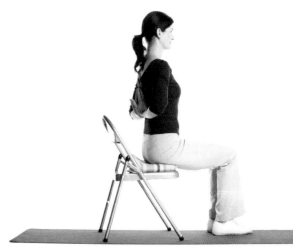

FIGURE 3A
REVERSE PRAYER POSE

Moving gently, and going only as far as feels comfortable, begin to press the fingertips upward toward your head, bringing the palms toward each other into a prayer position (Figure 3A). Stop whenever you feel that the stretch is enough for you, and breathe, keeping the chest lifted and open and the spine long and supported, lifting from the base of the spine and keeping the crown of the head directly over your tailbone.

You may feel this stretch primarily in the fingers, hands, and/or wrists, in which case you should be especially gentle and take care not to push. If the heels of the hands come closer together, you can press the hands more firmly, bringing the roots of the fingers together if possible. As you move deeper into the stretch in this manner, it is likely that you will feel more stretching sensation in the shoulders and chest. Either way, continue holding and breathing for 30 seconds to start with, working up to approximately 1 minute.

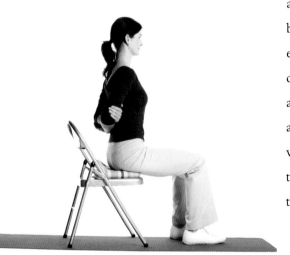

If this exercise feels painful or too difficult, an alternative is simply to fold your arms behind your back, trying to take hold of each elbow with the opposite hand (Figure 3B) or clasping each forearm with the opposite hand as close to your elbows as you can comfortably reach. Hold this position as in the first variation, with the chest lifted and open and the spine long, and repeat a second time with the arms crossed the opposite way.

FIGURE 3B
REVERSE PRAYER POSE, HOLDING ELBOWS

Seated Eagle Pose

GARUDASANA

▼ ▼ ▼ ▼ ▼ ▼ ▼ OPENS THE SHOULDER JOINTS AND UPPER BACK • RELEASES SHOULDER AND UPPER SPINE TENSION • STRETCHES THE ARMS AND WRISTS • FREES THE BREATH

CAUTIONS: Practice with care in the case of shoulder or upper back injuries.

PROP: 1 chair

OPTIONAL: 1 wedge or 1 blanket or 1 nonskid mat • 2nd nonskid mat

Begin in Seated Posture (Figure 1A or Figure 1B). Lengthen your spine, and stretch your arms out to your sides in a T position. We'll work in three stages.

Stage 1. Wrap your arms around your chest, as if you were giving yourself a hug, with the right arm on top of the left. Bring the hands around your shoulder blades, walking your fingertips toward your upper spine to the extent that is comfortable (Figure 4A).

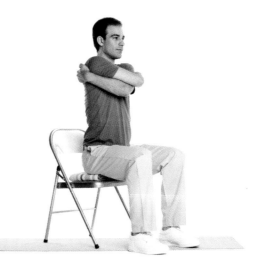

FIGURE 4A
SEATED EAGLE POSE, STAGE 1

Take a couple of relaxed, expansive breaths into your hands, so you feel the breath coming into the upper back and the area behind and between the shoulder blades becoming fuller and more open. If this feels like enough stretch in the upper back, it is fine to stop and hold here, breathing in to the thoracic spine and shoulder blade area for 30 seconds to 1 minute, and then releasing the arms. As this area opens up, you will likely be able to move to the next stage

Stage 2. If and when it is comfortable to move into a deeper stretch, bring the forearms and the backs of the hands toward each other, keeping the left elbow tucked firmly under the right. Stop when you feel a stretch in your upper back, and simply press the backs of the hands toward each other, or against one another if they are touching (Figure 4B).

Stage 3. Next, if the backs of the hands touch, and you are still comfortable to move a bit deeper, begin to wrap the arms. This is tricky, because intui-

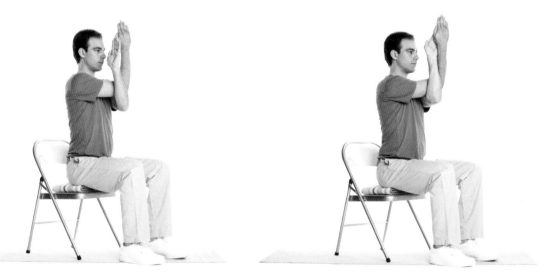

tively you will probably want to turn the hands, but instead keep the palms facing away from one another, and continue moving the hands toward and then past each other. The left hand should pass closer to your face as the hands move past one another. The hands continue to move away from each other and toward their opposite shoulders until the palms are facing one another. Once this is achieved, you can wrap the hands by pressing the left fingertips against the heel of the right hand. Then, with the shoulders still over the hips, lift the elbows up and out, away from the chest, and breathe into the upper back (Figure 4C).

Hold this stage for 30 seconds to 1 minute, breathing gently and feeling the upper back expand, the muscles around the upper spine and shoulder blades soften, and the shoulder blades themselves widen away from each other with each inhalation. Repeat on the other side, with the left arm on top of the right.

OPPOSITE:

FIGURE 4B
SEATED EAGLE POSE, STAGE 2

FIGURE 4C
SEATED EAGLE POSE, STAGE 3

Seated Cow Pose

GOMUKHASANA

▼ ▼ ▼ ▼ ▼ ▼ ▼ OPENS THE SHOULDER JOINTS AND CHEST
• STRETCHES THE MUSCLES OF THE SHOULDERS
AND ARMS • FREES THE BREATH

CAUTION: Practice with care in the case of shoulder injuries,
particularly rotator cuff injuries.

PROPS: 1 chair • 1 strap

OPTIONAL: 1 wedge or 1 blanket or 1 nonskid mat • 2nd nonskid mat

Begin in Seated Posture (Figure 1A or Figure 1B). Place a strap over your right
shoulder, letting one end drop down along your back. Lengthen your spine,
and stretch your arms out to your sides in a T position. Turn your arms away
from each other by internally rotating your left arm and externally rotating
your right. This means that your left palm will turn back and your right palm
will turn up, but the movement should initiate inside the shoulder joints, with
the hands following rather than leading. Continuing to rotate the arms in opposite directions, bring the right arm upward, stretching your fingertips toward
the ceiling while turning the palm toward your midline, and bring the left
arm down to your side, turning the palm backward. Once the arms are fully
stretched out in opposite directions, bend the elbows, dropping the left hand
behind your head and reaching down toward your upper back, and bringing

the right hand up your spine. As your hands reach toward each other, take hold of the strap from each end (Figure 5A).

You can walk the hands along the strap until you reach a comfortable level of stretch, and if the fingertips are able to touch comfortably, let go of the strap and clasp your hands instead, with your top hand turned palm in toward your back and your bottom hand turned outward (Figure 5B). Most people will need to use the strap to extend the reach of the arms, so don't strain to get your hands together; if they don't touch, continue to use the strap.

Hold this pose for 30 seconds to 1 minute, continuing to reach the elbows in opposite directions, feeling the shoulder muscles relax as you breathe. Release and place the strap over the left shoulder (if needed) to repeat on the opposite side.

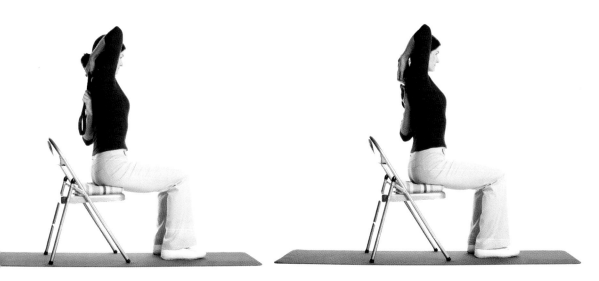

FIGURE 5A
SEATED COW POSE, WITH STRAP

FIGURE 5B
SEATED COW POSE

Seated Back Bend Pose

SALAMBA MAKARASANA

▼ ▼ ▼ ▼ ▼ ▼ STRETCHES THE MUSCLES OF ARMS, SHOULDERS, AND CHEST • RELEASES SHOULDER AND BACK TENSION • CREATES MOBILITY IN THE UPPER BACK • FREES THE BREATH • INCREASES ENERGY

CAUTIONS: Position your chair with the back against a wall or your desk, so it will not tip over backward if the front legs come off the floor! Practice with care in case of shoulder or neck injuries.

PROPS: 1 chair • 1 wall or a desk • 2 nonskid mats

OPTIONAL: 1 blanket • 1 block

Place your chair with the back at a wall, so it is stable. Fold one mat over the seat of the chair, so it is hanging over and padding the front edge, and spread the second mat on the floor, with the short edge just in front of the chair. Sitting on the mat on the floor, position yourself directly in front of the chair but facing away from it, so your upper spine rests against the chair seat. You want to place your upper, or thoracic, spine against the back of the chair, just above the lower tips of your shoulder blades; if you have a shorter spine, use a folded blanket under your sitting bones to elevate you to the right position. Clasp your hands behind your head, with your fingers interlaced and your elbows wide.

Begin by arching your spine over the seat of the chair, lifting up and over, rather than just leaning back, and rest your head in your hands as it comes back toward the seat of the chair. As you come deeper into the backbend, bring your elbows toward each other and reach them up toward the ceiling, so you are stretching upward from the sides of the chest and shoulders to the tips of the elbows. Be sure to keep the head supported in your hands, holding the base of your skull rather than your neck. Some people prefer to have more support for the head, so if your neck feels uncomfortable at all, place a block on the chair, and as your head drops backward, the block will be there to support it, with the hands resting against the block and the head resting in the palms of the hands. The block has three heights and can be adjusted for the amount of support that feels right for you. The important thing as you come into the backbend is to bend up and over the chair rather than simply leaning back against it; if you feel the front legs of the chair beginning to lift off the floor, you probably need to adjust your position so that the chair hits you a bit lower, allowing you to

FIGURE 6A
SEATED BACK BEND POSE

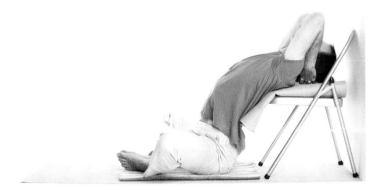

achieve this up-and-over action of the spine and chest, pressing slightly downward on the front edge of the chair seat as your spine bends over it. Once you feel this, bend back as far as feels comfortable and breathe, feeling your back muscles release and your chest expand and open. (Figure 6A).

For a more challenging variation, move from this pose into a deeper shoulder opener by keeping the spine in the same position, still resting your head back in your hands, but opening the elbows away from each other, stretching sideways from the shoulders to the tips of the elbows, as they reach away from each other and toward the sides of the room (Figure 6B). This version should be practiced very carefully and avoided altogether in the case of shoulder injuries.

Hold and breathe in this position for 30 seconds to 1 minute. To exit, keep the head supported, and use the arms to lift it back into an upright, seated position; then release the arms.

FIGURE 6B
SEATED BACK BEND POSE, ELBOWS OUT

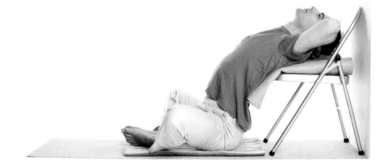

Seated Twist Pose

BHARADVAJASANA

▼ ▼ ▼ ▼ ▼ ▼ ▼ STRETCHES THE BACK MUSCLES
• EASES SHOULDER AND UPPER BACK TENSION • STRETCHES THE FRONT
AND SIDE TORSO • IMPROVES SEATED POSTURE AND BREATHING

CAUTIONS: Practice with care in case of shoulder or neck injuries.

PROP: 1 chair

OPTIONAL: a wall or desk • 1 wedge or 1 blanket
or 1 nonskid mat • 2nd nonskid mat

Sit sideways on your chair, with your right side facing the back of the chair.
You will be changing positions on the chair, so for added stability, placing the
chair back against a wall or your desk is a good option. If needed, position a
prop under your sitting bones to lift the pelvis, just as you would when facing
forward in Seated Posture (Figure 1A). Even if you don't require a lift under
your sitting bones to support your spine, a folded nonskid mat placed on the
seat is especially helpful for this pose, to keep your sitting bones from sliding
around on the chair as you twist. Place both feet firmly on the mat, hip-width
apart, with your heels directly under your knees, so the shins are perpendicular
to the floor. If you are using a mat on the floor to provide a pad for your feet,
position it so you can place your feet on it while sitting sideways.

Sit up tall, lengthening from the tailbone to the crown of the head, and take hold of the back of the chair with both hands, one hand holding each side of the chair's back. Maintaining a long spine and keeping your shoulders relaxed, gently turn your torso to the right (Figure 7). Use your hands to help guide the movement, but don't be forceful. Feel the twist beginning at the base of your spine and traveling, or spiraling, upward, so that the head is the last thing to turn, following, rather than leading, the movement. This movement should feel good, so stop when you reach a comfortable level of stretch and hold there, breathing naturally, for 30 seconds to 1 minute. As you hold the stretch, envision the spine becoming longer with each inhalation, and feel the body relaxing into the twisting position with each exhalation.

FIGURE 7
SEATED TWIST POSE

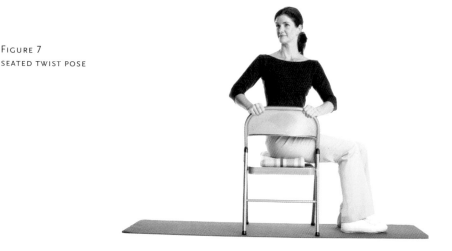

Release on an exhalation, turning the torso back in the direction of your knees. Once you have completely released from the twist and the spine is back to a neutral position, turn to the other side, and repeat in the opposite direction.

Seated Thread-the-Needle

▼ ▼ ▼ ▼ ▼ ▼ ▼ STRETCHES THE MUSCLES OF THE LOWER BACK
AND THE HIP ROTATORS • RELIEVES LOWER BACK TENSION
• HELPS WITH MOBILITY OF THE HIP SOCKETS AND HEALTHY POSTURE

CAUTION: Practice with care in case of lower back injuries.

PROP: 1 chair

OPTIONAL: a wall • 1 wedge or 1 blanket or 1 nonskid mat • 2nd nonskid mat

Begin in Seated Posture (Figure 1A or Figure 1B). You will be moving from an upright position to a forward bend, so if the chair feels like it might slip, placing your chair with the back against a wall or desk will add stability. We'll practice in two stages.

Stage 1. Once you are sitting up tall, in a healthy, comfortable position, with the feet firmly on the mat, hip-width apart and parallel to one another, lift out of the hip sockets. Bring the sacrum (the base of the spine) gently inward, toward the navel, and lengthen your spine to its full height. Then cross the right ankle over the left thigh, resting it in a flexed position just above the left knee. Place your hands on your hips and, keeping the front of your spine long and open and your right ankle flexed, begin to lean forward (Figure 8A). Your neck should also stay long, and your head should stay in a neutral position, continuing the line of the spine, rather than lifting or dropping from the shoulders. Still keeping the right ankle flexed, allow your right thigh to relax, dropping into the pull of gravity. However, don't push the thigh or knee toward the floor. Instead, simply let the thighbone relax in the hip socket and allow gravity to do the work of releasing the hip, as you continue to lengthen forward from the hip sockets. Breathe deeply, as you feel the muscles releasing around the right hip joint.

This first stage may feel quite intense, especially to start with, in which case it is enough to do until the hip muscles release a bit more. Don't go to the next stage until the first one is comfortable. If this stage feels like enough, hold here for 30 seconds to 1 minute. To come out, simply lift the torso back to an upright position, still keeping the spine long and the head and neck neutral as you come up. Once your torso is upright, place your right hand under your right knee and lift the knee toward you before uncrossing the legs.

Stage 2. When you are ready, the next stage is to relax your arms over your right shin and drop them toward the floor (Figure 8B). Then drop your head, and allow your spine to relax downward as well. Do this only after you have

FIGURE 8A
SEATED THREAD-THE-NEEDLE, STAGE 1

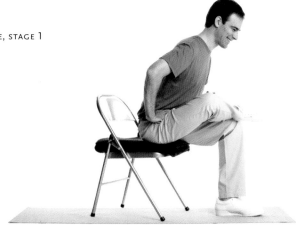

lengthened forward through the front spine to the maximum that is comfortable; the forward movement is the more important one. As you release the spine in this second stage, you add more weight and gravity to the hip stretch, and you will feel the sensation increase. Stay at an intensity level that feels reasonable to you; consistency (regular stretching) is more important than how far you go in any particular stretch, and you need to be able to relax in a stretching position to get the full benefit from it.

Hold the pose, breathing naturally, for 30 seconds to 1 minute, working up to 2 minutes as your comfort level allows. To come out of this second stage, keep your head and neck relaxed as you bring your hands back to the hips. Press into the floor with your left foot, and lengthen the spine forward as you come up to a full sitting position, leading with the sternum. Once the spine is upright, place your right hand under your right knee and lift it away from the floor. As the knee comes up, supported by your hand, it is safe and easy to uncross the leg and place the foot back on the floor. Repeat on the second side.

FIGURE 8B
SEATED THREAD-THE-NEEDLE, STAGE 2

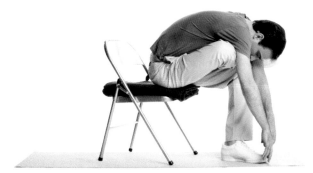

Standing Forward Bend Pose

EKA PADA SALAMBA UTTANASANA

▼ ▼ ▼ ▼ ▼ ▼ ▼ STRETCHES THE MUSCLES OF THE SPINE AND THE HIP ROTATORS • RELIEVES BACK AND NECK TENSION • HELPS WITH MOBILITY OF THE HIP SOCKETS AND HEALTHY POSTURE

CAUTION: Practice with care in case of lower back injuries.

PROP: 1 chair

OPTIONAL: a wall • 1 or 2 nonskid mats

Stand facing the side of the chair seat. You will be changing positions on the chair, so for added stability, you can place the back of your chair against a wall. For even more stability, try placing one nonskid mat under the chair and a folded nonskid mat on the chair seat. If you are practicing at the wall, rest your right hand on it for balance.

Step your right foot forward and up onto the seat. The toes of both feet should be facing the same direction you are, rather than turning in or out. Once you are balanced with your right foot on the chair, press firmly into both feet and then lean forward and bend over, letting your spine hang down inside the right thigh and your head drop toward the floor in a deep forward bend (Figure 9). Keep your hips in line with the standing leg and your weight balanced evenly between the front and back of the standing foot, rather than leaning back and resting your weight on your heel. Press into the foot on the chair, and relax from the stretching hip, allowing gravity to stretch the muscles of the pelvis and the back.

If it is comfortable, both arms can dangle down toward the floor, increasing the stretch in the back, shoulders, and neck. If the stretch is too intense or balance feels a bit shaky, instead place your right hand on the chair inside the foot; this will both reduce the stretch and help with stability. In either case, let go of the weight of your head and feel the release of the neck muscles as you breathe gently and naturally.

Hold for 30 seconds to 1 minute. To come out, bend the standing knee, and roll your spine back up to standing, one vertebrae at a time, with the arms still dangling and the head coming up last. Once your head is upright again, straighten the standing leg, and roll the shoulders down and back. When you feel fully balanced, step back down to the floor, and move to the other side of the chair, turning around to repeat on the second side.

FIGURE 9
STANDING FORWARD BEND POSE

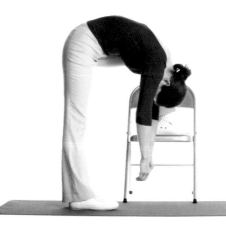

Seated Forward Bend Pose

SALAMBA UTTANASANA

▼ ▼ ▼ ▼ ▼ ▼ ▼ STRETCHES THE MUSCLES OF THE SPINE AND
PELVIS • RELIEVES BACK AND NECK TENSION • HELPS WITH
MOBILITY OF THE HIP SOCKETS AND HEALTHY POSTURE

CAUTION: Practice with care in case of lower back injuries.

PROP: 1 chair

OPTIONAL: a wall or desk • 1 wedge or 1 blanket
or 1 nonskid mat • 2nd nonskid mat • 2 blocks

Sit down, facing forward, in Seated Posture (Figure 1A or Figure 1B). For extra stability, you can place your chair with the back against a wall or desk.

Place your feet firmly on the floor, slightly wider than your hips, so they are just outside the legs of the chair. With your knees directly over your heels, turn your toes just slightly outward. Place your hands on your legs mid-thigh and stretch forward, lengthening the front of your spine and stretching the crown of your head out in front of you. Then, pressing into your feet, relax your spine, dropping your head toward the floor and letting your rib cage and arms release down between your legs (Figure 10). If your hands reach the floor, just let them rest there, keeping the neck, shoulders, and elbows completely relaxed. If your hands do not easily reach the floor, place blocks under your hands, shoulder-width apart, so that your back has some support from below as you relax your shoulders, arms, and hands. Keep pressing your feet into the floor for balance, and relax from the hip sockets, breathing gently and naturally.

FIGURE 10
SEATED FORWARD BEND POSE

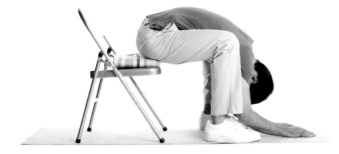

Hold this pose for at least 30 seconds, up to 2 minutes. To come out, keep your neck and head relaxed as you replace your hands onto the legs. Make sure your hands are on the center of the thighbones, to avoid pushing on the knees. Press into your hands and feet to lift yourself back up to sitting, letting the neck stay soft and with the head following, rather than leading, the movement.

This stretch should feel good. It can be repeated often throughout the day.

Seated Neck Stretches

▼ ▼ ▼ ▼ ▼ ▼ ▼ STRETCHES THE MUSCLES OF THE NECK,
SHOULDERS, AND UPPER BACK • RELIEVES NECK AND SHOULDER
TENSION • HELPS WITH HEADACHES

CAUTION: Practice carefully in case of neck injuries.

PROP: 1 chair

OPTIONAL: 1 wedge or 1 blanket or 1 nonskid mat • 2nd nonskid mat

Side Neck Stretch. Sit in Seated Posture (Figure 1A or Figure 1B). Maintaining a long, supported spine and facing forward, relax your neck and let your head

LEFT TO RIGHT:

FIGURE 11A
SIDE NECK STRETCH

FIGURE 11B
SIDE NECK STRETCH, ARMS AT SIDES

FIGURE 11C
SIDE NECK STRETCH, ARM DRAPED
OVER THE HEAD

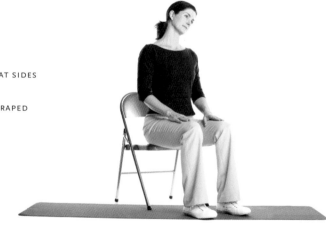

drop to the right, as if you were going to drop your right ear onto your right shoulder (Figure 11A). Keep your shoulders relaxed and your chest lifted and open, and let the weight of your head stretch out the muscles along the left side of your neck and the top of your shoulder, as your head continues to relax to the right.

If the weight of your head gives you a good feeling of stretch, keep your hands placed gently on your legs. For a deeper stretch, your arms can drop down to your sides and hang from your shoulders (Figure 11B). For even more, keep your right arm dropped but lift your left arm and drape it over the right side of the head, to give the stretch a little more weight (Figure 11C).

A few cautions to keep in mind if you choose this last option: Keep the left shoulder relaxed, taking care not to squeeze or lift the shoulder muscles as you lift the arm; keep the chest lifted and the spine centered and upright, rather than pulling yourself toward the right; and, most important, do not pull on the neck

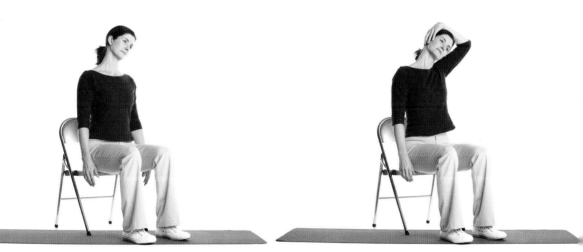

with the arm, but rather just let the arm rest lightly on the side of the head. For best results, press the side of the head and the arm gently against one another. This is known as an isometric stretch.

Hold the stretch from 30 seconds to 1 minute, breathing with awareness and feeling the stretching muscles release. The neck is delicate, so be especially sensitive when stretching neck muscles; it should always feel like a welcome amount of stretching sensation and not overly intense. To come out, first drop the arm if you have lifted it. Keep the face forward as you lift the head back up to center, as if your right ear was pulling it back up. Wait until the neck feels relaxed and neutral again before repeating this stretch to the second side.

Forward Neck Stretch. After you have stretched both sides, you can also stretch the back of the neck by dropping the head forward, resting your chin toward your chest (Figure 11D). Again, keep your spine long and your chest lifted and open as you do this. When you drop the head, you will feel a stretch

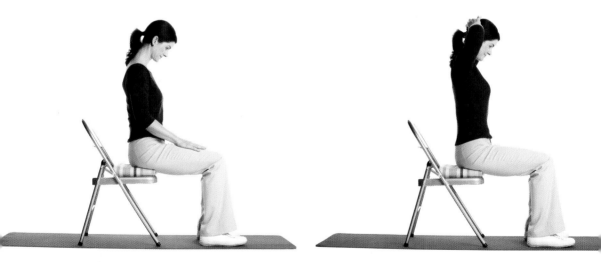

along the back of your neck and probably along your upper back as well. If you feel a good stretch from the weight of your head, you are doing enough and should again keep the arms relaxed. To deepen the stretch in this phase of full neck flexion, place the hands lightly on the back of the skull, interlacing the fingers (Figure 11E). Make sure your hands are on your skull, not your neck, and keep the elbows wide and stretching outward to the sides, rather than dropping toward the floor. Avoid pulling on the neck; again, you can press the back of the head and the hands isometrically together. Breathe into your upper back, as you hold this stretch for 30 seconds to 1 minute.

To come out, first drop your hands back to your lap, if you have placed them behind your head. Then lift the head back up gently. You can press slightly into your hands, but keep your arms and shoulder relaxed, and continue looking downward as the back of your skull draws up. When the head is upright, stay seated for a few moments, still breathing gently and with awareness, until the neck feels relaxed and neutral again. It may help to move the head around very lightly, both up and down and side to side (as if you were very gently shaking your head yes and no).

OPPOSITE:

FIGURE 11D
FORWARD NECK STRETCH

FIGURE 11E
FORWARD NECK STRETCH, FINGERS INTERLACED

Seated Lion Pose

▼ ▼ ▼ ▼ ▼ ▼ ▼ STRETCHES THE FACE AND JAW • IMPROVES
BREATHING AND ENERGY • HELPS WITH HEADACHES

CAUTION: If you don't have a private workspace,
this asana might be more comfortably practiced at home.

PROP: 1 chair

OPTIONAL: 1 wedge or 1 blanket or 1 nonskid mat • 2nd nonskid mat

Begin in Seated Posture (Figure 1A or Figure 1B). Relax your face, closing your
eyes if you would like, and letting your breath relax as well.

Place your hands on your knees and, keeping your spine straight, lean slightly
forward and lift up through your chest, straightening your arms and gently
arching the back. Let the head tilt upward, but do not squeeze or shorten the
back of the neck; keep a sense of space at the base of the skull where it meets
the spine.

As you lift through the head and chest, let your eyes open and look down
to gaze lightly at the tip of your nose. Take a deep inhalation through your
nose. Then open your mouth as wide as you can and stick your tongue out and
stretch it toward your chin (Figure 12). As you exhale through your mouth, let
go with whatever sound wants to come out. This is the roar of the lion.

Repeat this exercise 3 to 5 times, letting the sound become a bit louder each time. The wider you open your mouth and the farther you stick out your tongue, the greater the release. Although it may seem silly at first, you will notice feeling refreshed afterward. This exercise is a great way to relieve both muscle tension and mental stress. Notice how much more relaxed the muscles of the face and jaw feel following Lion Pose; even if you weren't previously aware of holding tension there, you will definitely feel a difference as it begins to release.

After the last repetition, relax your arms and face, and let the spine come back to a neutral position, with the crown of your head placed directly above the tailbone. Let your breathing relax back to a natural rhythm, and sit quietly for a few moments before moving on to the next exercise or asana or returning to work.

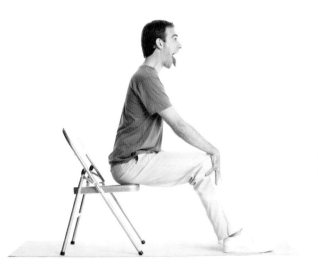

FIGURE 12
SEATED LION POSE

Chair Dog Pose

SALAMBA ADHO MUKHA SVANASANA

▼ ▼ ▼ ▼ ▼ ▼ ▼ STRETCHES THE MUSCLES OF THE LEGS, BACK, AND SHOULDERS • RELEASES SHOULDER AND BACK TENSION • CREATES MOBILITY IN THE HIP SOCKETS NECESSARY TO SUPPORT HEALTHY SEATED POSTURE

CAUTIONS: Practice with care in case of hamstring, lower back, or shoulder injuries.

PROPS: 1 chair • 1 wall or desk

OPTIONAL: 2 nonskid mats

For stability, place the back of your chair against a wall or desk. Some people prefer to use a mat for this pose and others like to practice it on the bare floor, especially if wearing shoes. If you choose to use a mat, place it in front of the chair, with the short end facing the chair. Either way, you can remove your shoes for comfort.

Stand in front of the chair and bend forward, placing your hands at the front edge of the chair seat, palms flat. If the chair is slippery, or if you experience discomfort in your wrists, placing a folded nonskid mat on the seat of the chair may help. To help reduce sensation in the wrists, place the heels of your hands at the edge of the folded mat, so they are higher than the fingers; this creates a lesser angle for the wrist joints.

With your feet hip-width apart, step back until your arms are straight and your heels are under or slightly behind your hips, depending on what feels best. As you lengthen your spine, keep your heels grounded and your neck relaxed, with your head placed comfortably between your arms (Figure 13). Hold this stretch for 30 seconds to 1 minute, breathing gently, as you press your thigh-bones gently back against your hamstrings, draw your hips up and back, away from your hands, and stretch your tailbone away from the crown of your head. To exit, walk toward the chair before standing up.

You can practice this stretch often throughout the day. You may feel it in your shoulders and the sides of your chest as well as in your hamstring and calf muscles. If you are very stiff in the hamstrings, especially if you are tall, you may find it better to turn the chair around and use its back for support, rather than the seat, or use your desk instead of a chair. You want to find the right height for your body proportions and flexibility.

FIGURE 13
CHAIR DOG POSE

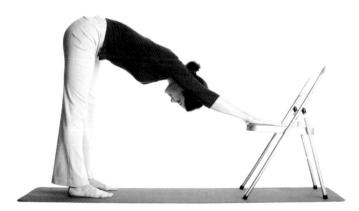

Inverted Legs Relaxation Pose

VIPARITA KARANI

▼ ▼ ▼ ▼ ▼ ▼ ▼ IMPROVES THE CIRCULATORY, NERVOUS, AND
IMMUNE SYSTEMS • RELAXES THE MUSCLES OF THE LOWER BACK
• REDUCES STRESS • INCREASES MENTAL CLARITY AND ALERTNESS

CAUTIONS: Do not practice this pose if it is painful for your lower back
or past the seventeenth week of pregnancy. Menstruating women
should practice the chair version.

PROPS: 1 nonskid mat • 1 chair or a wall • 1 or 2 blankets
• 1 pillow • a timer

OPTIONAL: 1 wedge

Hopefully you will feel peaceful and relaxed following this pose. The challenge is to maintain some of this feeling as you go back to your computer!

With a chair. Place your mat in front of your chair, with the short end of the mat facing the chair. Spread your blanket on top of your mat, if you would like more padding underneath your spine when you are lying down. Fold the second blanket in half and have it nearby. Set a timer for the length of time that you want to relax: at least 5 minutes and ideally 10 to 15.

Lie down on the mat on your back, with your sitting bones close to the chair and your calves resting on the seat of the chair. Bring the chair close to you, so the backs of the knees are fully supported on the edge of the chair seat. Place a firm pillow under your neck and head for support. Relax your arms, with your hands either resting on your rib cage or on the floor at your sides, palms facing up, whichever feels most comfortable (Figure 14A). This position is generally very soothing and comfortable for the lower back, but if you have a back condition or injury that causes discomfort here, it may be alleviated by placing a wedge under your sacrum, with the thin edge pointed toward your torso, so your tailbone is supported on the thicker edge and is thus tipped upward toward your knees Once you are comfortable, close your eyes.

As you let the weight of your body relax into the floor, bring your awareness to your breath. Observing your breath, as in Breathing Awareness (see page 68), will help you both relax and focus. As you relax, you can gradually let go of watching your breath and let your mind empty. But if this is difficult, periodically bring the mind back to your breath, so it doesn't drift or race off with your thoughts.

FIGURE 14A
INVERTED LEGS RELAXATION POSE, WITH A CHAIR

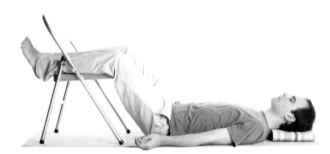

When the timer goes off, if you are ready to come out, wait for an inhalation and, with it, bring your knees toward your chest. Hug your legs gently into your body, and pause there for a few more breath cycles. Then, with an exhalation, turn over to one side and again pause there for a few more quiet moments. When you feel ready, press yourself up, using the support of one or both arms, letting your head be the last thing to come up. Looking down at the floor will help prevent you from leading with your head and neck.

At the wall. In this version, you use the wall instead of a chair. Place your mat perpendicular to the wall, and spread a blanket on your mat for extra padding, if desired. Fold the second blanket into thirds or use a firm pillow, and place it toward the end of the mat, 1 or 2 inches away from the wall. Set a timer for the length of time you want to relax.

Sit sideways on your pillow or folded blanket, with one side facing the wall. You will be sliding sideways onto your back to bring your legs up onto the wall and rest your low back on the support of the pillow. This can be awkward at first and takes a bit of learning, but it will become easy with practice. Begin by leaning back toward the floor while pressing the side of your hip as close to the wall as possible. As you come backward onto your elbows, begin to pivot your pelvis, staying as close to the wall as you can while you move, and swinging your legs around to rest on the wall, straight up from the pillow. As you do this, your head can come to rest on your mat (Figure 14B).

Your sitting bones do not need to be touching the wall. Comfort is the key to this pose, and you can move as far from the wall as feels good for your body, perhaps just resting your heels on the wall rather than the entirety of the legs. What is more important is that you not feel like you are sliding off the pillow or blanket toward your head. Make sure that your lower back is firmly supported, and allow your tailbone to drop slightly over the edge of the pillow, toward the wall. Adjust your distance from the wall so you are close enough that your low back is comfortable but far enough away that there is little or no sensation or stretch in your hamstrings. If the hamstring stretch increases as you hold the pose, move yourself a little farther from the wall so you remain comfortable and relaxed. The objective of this asana is to release and relax, so as far as possible you want to eliminate distractions, including the sensation of stretching muscles. In cases of low back discomfort, remove the blanket and rest the back flat on the floor instead of lifting the pelvis. If more support is needed to make the low back comfortable, use the wedge, as described in the chair version. Find a very comfortable, relaxed position in this pose, and then close your eyes and proceed as for the chair version.

FIGURE 14B
INVERTED LEGS RELAXATION POSE, AT THE WALL

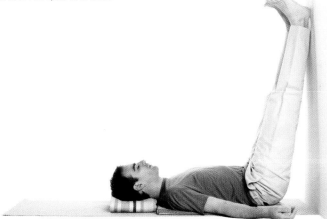

Breathing Awareness and Meditation

▼ ▼ ▼ ▼ ▼ ▼ ▼ REDUCES STRESS AND ANXIETY • IMPROVES
BREATHING, ENERGY, AND MENTAL CLARITY

CAUTIONS: Practice with care in cases of anxiety or depression;
cease practice if anxiety arises or increases.

PROP: 1 chair or 1 nonskid mat

OPTIONAL: 1 wedge or 1 blanket or 1 nonskid mat • 2nd nonskid mat
• 2 blocks or blankets • a wall • a timer

You can practice this exercise either in Seated Posture (Figure 15A) or, if it is
comfortable, sitting on the floor in Bound Angle Pose (Figure 15B) or in any
cross-legged position that feels easy. (See pages 31 and 94 for instructions on
how to practice the poses as pictured.)

Whatever position you choose, make sure it is comfortable for both your
back and your knees. If you are on the floor, placing a wedge or a firmly folded
blanket or a folded nonskid mat under your sitting bones may help with this,
just as it does with Seated Posture; and blocks or folded blankets placed under
each knee may also make a sitting on the floor more comfortable. It is also fine
to use a wall to support your back, as long as you are sitting close enough to
the wall to avoid slumping against it.

Whether on a chair or the floor, sit with a long spine, and place your hands on your thighs, allowing your arms and shoulders to relax and drop. Check your alignment: your shoulders should be directly over your hips and the crown of your head over your tailbone. Once you feel balanced and aligned, close your eyes, maintaining a long spine as you relax from the inside. Close your mouth and relax your face, breathing through your nose.

Breathing Awareness. Bring your awareness inward, and let your mind begin to relax and focus on your breath. At first, don't do anything to change or control your breath, but simply tune in with awareness and observe the breath as it flows naturally in and out. This is often more challenging than it sounds, as the mind is built to think and tends to wander off with your thoughts. Learning to keep your attention on your breath is a kind of mental training that takes

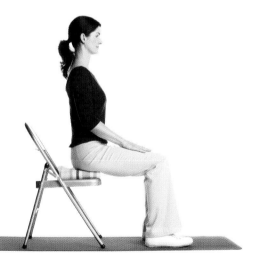

FIGURE 15A
BREATHING AWARENESS IN SEATED POSTURE

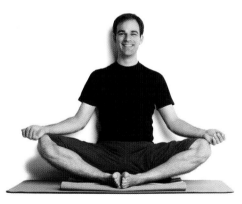

FIGURE 15B
BREATHING AWARENESS IN BOUND ANGLE POSE

practice, but with it comes the benefit of increased focus and clarity. So each time you notice your mind drifting away from the breath, gently bring it back. Be kind with yourself, no matter how many times this occurs. This is both the lesson and the practice of mindfulness.

As you become more practiced at observing your breath, a helpful tool is to place the hands on the body to direct the breath into different areas. This helps to open the lungs for increased breath capacity and also gives the mind a specific task to focus on, increasing the concentration aspect of the exercise. As you place your hands on your belly, you can send the breath down into the lower portion of the lungs and feel the abdomen gently expand and release for a few breaths. Then place your hands on your low back. The back body often doesn't receive as much breath, and the sensations and movements may feel unfamiliar as you send the breath there. Then move your hands to your side rib cage, and feel the lungs broaden outward from the spine, as the breath moves into the side body and the middle portion of the lungs. See if you can sense your diaphragm, just behind the solar plexus (where the floating ribs come together below the chest), receiving breath as well. Next fold your arms across your chest and place the hands on the sides of your chest, inside your upper arms. As you move the breath into your hands, you will feel the breath moving higher into the lungs, continuing to open into the side body but also expanding into the upper back, behind and between your shoulder blades. Finally, rest your fingertips on your upper chest, just below the collarbones, and feel the breath come into the highest area of the lungs, sensing where they connect at the clavicles, as you gently direct the breath into your touch.

Stay with each stage for at least 1 or 2 minutes, and observe which areas your breath flows to easily and naturally and which places feel more constricted or resistant to receiving the breath—which paths, in other words, are less traveled by the respiratory system. According to Dennis Lewis, author of *The Tao of Natural Breathing,* the human lung capacity is approximately 5,000 milliliters, but the average amount of air in each breath we take is just 500! So for most of us, many areas of the lungs, and the corresponding muscles that support them, are underused. It is quite typical to breathe habitually into either the belly or the chest, neglecting the other portions of the lungs, and those with voice or musical training may have been taught diaphragmatic breathing techniques. One of the benefits of asana is to open up the underused areas and naturally increase the amount of breath capacity we use. This is one of the fundamental reasons that practicing yoga is energizing: Physiologically yoga actually increases the amount of oxygen our cells receive with each breath. While it is healthful to increase our oxygen intake, this should happen gradually, over time, because the body can integrate only so much change at one time. As new areas of the lungs open more fully, you may experience some stretching sensation in the surrounding muscle tissue, but this should feel welcome and pleasant rather than intense or painful. So don't strain or push as you do this exercise; continue to breathe gently, and aim for a comfortable, rather than maximum, level of expansion of the lungs.

This whole exercise can be done in less than 10 minutes, although it is fine to take longer, as long as it is comfortable both physically and mentally. If you find yourself becoming tense or anxious, it is better to let go of trying to control your breath and move back to simply observing, or come out of it altogether. Once you have finished exploring opening the different areas of the lungs, rest your hands back onto your lap, allow the breath to relax into its natural state, and resume quietly observing your breath for another few minutes. Depending on how you feel, this exercise can either end here, or you can move into a final stage of meditation for a few more minutes.

Meditation. Breathing Awareness is an introduction to pranayama, which works with learning to consciously control the breath. Pranayama also serves to prepare the nervous system and the mind for meditation. As you practice observing your breath, the nervous system moves into its more relaxed, parasympathetic mode, and you are training the mind to focus in a particular way, to become simultaneously both quieter and more aware. The next step is to move from breath-focused meditation to general meditation, or *dhyana*. Although there are numerous and varying approaches to meditation, the intention of virtually all of them is to learn to be more fully present in the moment.

To begin practicing basic meditation, simply move your attention from your breath to watching the activity of your mind. Meditation is often defined as "emptying the mind," but, rather than trying to close your mind or shut out your thoughts, it is usually more effective to open your mind and observe the thoughts that come into it as part of its natural process, creating a general sense of awareness. The trick is learning to observe the thoughts and let them go again, very much as you previously observed and released each breath. Watching your thoughts as they pass through instead of getting caught up with them is what makes this meditation rather than thinking. As you practice this technique, anything you notice about what you are feeling in the moment is part of the meditative process. The idea is to be present and observe your moment-to-moment experience, accepting the mind's response as part of the experience and resisting the urge to move into judging or analyzing it. This is not a state that comes naturally to the human brain, and it usually requires a great deal of practice. Start with just 2 or 3 minutes, and work up to longer periods of time, as you feel ready. Studies show that a 10- to 20-minute session of meditation, when practiced regularly, can have profound mental and physiological benefits.

Whenever you are ready to stop, first bring your attention back to your body, and notice how you are feeling physically. You want to be grounded following meditation, so notice particularly the touch of your feet on the floor and your sitting bones on your chair or the floor, and gently press downward through both to create firmer contact with the ground. Once you are ready, simply open your eyes. Then sit quietly for a few moments and take your time before going back to your computer. When you do, see if you can maintain the quiet, mindful energy of meditation, and see how that affects your feeling of well-being, and possibly even your productivity, as you go about your day.

Setting a timer for these exercises will help you keep track of time and allow you to keep your eyes closed until you are ready to move out of meditation. Try to make at least a few minutes of breathing and meditation part of your regular daily routine. Although it can be difficult to make "doing nothing" a priority, our brains and bodies desperately need this nondoing time on a regular basis to stay healthy. A meditation practice is a step toward regaining balance in your life, and there are great health benefits to allowing the nervous system to relax deeply, including a fortified immune system. Increased breath capacity translates to increased energy, and you should feel both refreshed and relaxed after these practices.

Part Three

Computer-Free Yoga

▼ ▼ ▼ ▼ ▼ ▼ ▼ ▼ ▼ ▼ ▼

Dedicated Yoga Practice for People Who Spend Long Hours at Their Computers

IN ADDITION TO the stretching breaks you take during your workday or computer time, a well-rounded yoga program includes some dedicated practice, completely away from the computer. A dedicated home practice gives you more privacy and flexibility, allowing you to include more asanas, which can round out your practice. Although you can do yoga whenever you can find or make a few free moments, ideal times for personal practice are first thing in the morning or following other types of exercise and at the end of the day, as you transition from work to home. This applies even if you work at home; your yoga practice can provide an effective and healthy shift between work mode and your nonworking hours.

The great benefit of practicing when you first get up in the morning is that it sets you up for a focused, energetic day. Following a morning yoga session, your mind will be clearer and possibly even more productive, and your breath will be freer and fuller, which is both energizing and relaxing. One thing we learn from yoga is that energy and relaxation are complementary rather than contradictory, and together they create a balanced state of being. Most of all, you will be more aware in your body, more likely to make natural ergonomic adjustments (those that maximize comfort and safety as you sit at your computer) without much conscious effort, and more liable to notice when you need to take a break and do some countermovements to stay in balance. Also, first thing in the morning your stomach is empty, which is ideal for yoga. While most of the exercises in this book do not require a completely empty stomach, it is always easier on the body to exercise when energy is not being diverted to the digestive system, and a deeper yoga practice does include exercises that are best not performed after eating. Practicing before breakfast can also help to improve digestion and metabolism.

If you are including other forms of exercise in your self-care program (and it is great if you are, the more variety the better), another excellent time to incorporate some yoga into your life is immediately following your run, swim, bicycle ride, or hang-gliding session. Stretching your muscles when they are still warm from vigorous use is important and beneficial for several reasons. First, it will help prevent them from becoming overly tight as a result of the repetitive contraction inherent in virtually all forms of aerobic exercise. Supple, balanced muscles don't pull as hard on the skeleton, which keeps the joints balanced and far less prone to injury. Second, warm muscles stretch more easily and more fully, so this is the ideal time to work on improving your range of motion; delaying your after-workout stretching until a later yoga practice is not nearly as effective in this regard. Last, following a strenuous workout with stretching and relaxation creates an optimum physical experience for a healthy, balanced body and nervous system.

Yoga practice also makes for a wonderful transition from work to home, or even between work-related computer time and personal Web surfing. Often we have habits or even addictions that help us wind down at the end of the day. Establishing the routine of a short yoga or relaxation session to help fulfill this function—before we reach for that glass of wine or bag of chips or remote control—can reduce or even eliminate the need for those crutches and give us the option of choosing more freely how we satisfy our needs. Even five minutes of meditation or one of the relaxation poses (such as Inverted Legs Relaxation Pose or Letting Go Pose) can help ease us out of work mode and into our personal life. Add a few stretches beforehand, and you may find that you are able to move into the evening feeling more refreshed and fully present.

More Poses: Away from the Computer

Standing Side-Stretch Pose

ARDHA URDHVA HASTASANA

▼ ▼ ▼ ▼ ▼ ▼ ▼ OPENS SHOULDERS AND RELIEVES SHOULDER
TENSION • STRETCHES INTERCOSTAL MUSCLES • IMPROVES
BREATHING AND ENERGY

CAUTION: Practice with care in case of shoulder injuries.

PROP: a wall

OPTIONAL: 1 nonskid mat

Stand with your right side facing the wall, feet close to each other and parallel to one another, and your right foot just a few inches from the wall. Many people like to use a mat for standing poses, rather than standing on carpet or a bare floor; if you prefer a mat, place the short end against the wall. Lean into the wall with your right hip, and stretch your right arm up along the wall, leaning your whole right side into the wall, from your hip to your fingertips. Keep the arm alongside your ear or a little in front of it as you reach it up the wall, rather than letting it drift back behind your head. For more stretch, you can turn your chest slightly away from the wall and your stretching arm toward your left shoulder.

Start by firmly pressing your feet into the floor and lengthening up through your side body from your hip to your fingertips, possibly crawling the fingertips farther up the wall. Stay gentle with this action, as the stretch will increase quite a bit as you move through the next stages of this exercise. Next, keeping your right side in contact with the wall, begin to lift your heels off the floor, allowing your rib cage and your arm to slide up along the wall as you lift high onto the balls of your feet, like a dancer (Figure 16). Continue to reach through the fingertips as your arm slides up the wall, again crawling the fingertips upward if it feels comfortable. Hold this lift for a few moments, breathing gently into your stretching side and feeling the ribs and the side of the chest lengthening and opening.

Then, as you begin to lower your heels slowly back onto the floor, try to keep your arm high on the wall. Don't overdo this, as you will be getting a big stretch in the intercostal muscles and side of the chest, but do gently resist letting the arm slide down with you. Once your feet are firmly back on the floor, again press into them and lengthen up through the fingertips, still leaning into the wall. Hold for a few more breaths, as you feel the muscles along the side of the body softening and releasing and your breath moving more fully into the stretching side. To come out, slide your arm down along the wall in front of you. Then turn around and repeat on the other side.

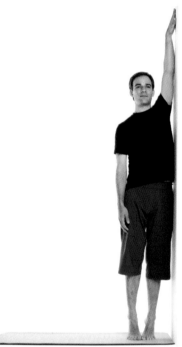

FIGURE 16
STANDING SIDE STRETCH POSE

Supported Spine-Stretch Pose

SALAMBA ADHO MUKHA SVANASANA

▼ ▼ ▼ ▼ ▼ ▼ ▼ STRETCHES THE WHOLE BODY • RELIEVES LOWER
BACK AND SHOULDER TENSION • INCREASES ENERGY

CAUTIONS: Practice with care in case of hamstring, lower back, or shoulder injuries.

PROP: a table or counter or kitchen sink

OPTIONAL: 1 nonskid mat

This pose is similar to Chair Dog Pose (Figure 13), but with the arms placed higher in relation to the pelvis, so that most or all of your weight stays with your legs. You can experiment with finding the right height to support your pose, and even work with the arms placed at or above the level of the pelvis, rather than below. A table may work for you, or a kitchen counter (or bookshelf or something else about that height) may work better, depending on your height and proportions, as well as your flexibility. Again, you are looking to rest your hands at about the level of your front hipbones, or slightly higher. Make sure that whatever you are using is stable and will not to slide away from you; brace it against the wall if you need to.

Stand in front of the table, with your feet hip-width apart and parallel to one another. If you prefer to stand on a mat, place it perpendicular to the table, with the short end facing it. Place your hands on the table, palms down, and then step back with both feet, dropping your chest and walking back until your arms are straight, your heels are under your hip sockets, and your spine is approximately parallel with the floor. If the support for your hands is higher than your front hip bones, your arms and shoulders will also end up higher than the pelvis, in which case the spine will not be exactly parallel to the floor. This is okay and may actually be preferable if you have tight hamstrings; as long as you can straighten your arms and extend your spine fully, it is fine to stretch wider than a 90-degree angle. Create an angle that your hamstrings are comfortable with; don't overdo.

Keep your head in neutral between your arms, with your feet pressing firmly into the floor, still parallel to one another, and hip-width apart (Figure 17). Lengthen backward through your spine, thinking of uncurling your tailbone as you stretch it away from the crown of your head. As you stretch fully through your spine, try to keep your rib cage centered in your body, taking care not to overarch or sag in the low back.

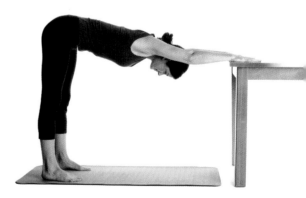

Although a major benefit of this stretch is to create more space between the vertebrae and reduce compression in the low back, it is a full body stretch, and you may feel it elsewhere in the body, depending on where you are tight, including the hamstrings and the shoulder joints (especially the armpits and sides of the chest). Breathe naturally and easily in this stretch for 30 seconds to 1 minute, and eventually up to 2 minutes. To come out, keep your hands on the table to support your back as you walk forward, so you are supported until you are standing fully upright again.

For a variation on this basic stretch, I like to use my kitchen sink, because I can grab hold of it as I walk my feet back and lengthen my spine. This version creates a bit more traction for the spine and the shoulder joints, as the spine hangs back away from the sink. If you try this version, as you feel your muscles loosen up, you can create yet more traction by walking your feet slightly forward of your hip sockets and allowing your pelvis and tailbone to hang back behind your feet a bit. You can do this for an extra stretch anytime you are in your kitchen!

OPPOSITE:
FIGURE 17
SUPPORTED SPINE-STRETCH POSE

Supported Shoulder-Stretch Pose

SALAMBA ARDHA ADHO MUKHA SVANASANA

▼ ▼ ▼ ▼ ▼ ▼ ▼ STRETCHES THE MUSCLES OF THE SPINE AND
SHOULDERS • RELIEVES UPPER BACK AND SHOULDER TENSION • OPENS
THE UPPER BACK AND IMPROVES BREATHING

CAUTIONS: Practice with care in case of hamstring, lower back, or shoulder injuries.

PROP: 1 table or counter

OPTIONAL: 1 or 2 nonskid mats • 1 towel • 1 block

Stand in front of your table or counter. As in Supported Spine-Stretch Pose, you are looking for a height that is at or above the level of your front hipbones. If you prefer to stand on a mat, place it with the short end facing the table. Position your elbows at the edge, shoulder-width apart, and bring your hands together, with the palms pressing against one another and your fingertips facing upward, in Prayer Pose.

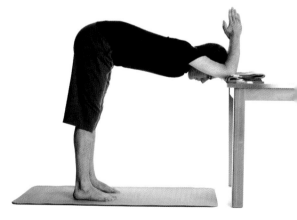

FIGURE 18A
SUPPORTED SHOULDER-STRETCH POSE

If you like, you can use a folded towel or a folded nonskid mat under your elbows, to cushion the table.

Keeping your elbows in position on the table, begin to walk back, as in Supported Spine-Stretch Pose, dropping your chest and lengthening your spine backward, until your heels are under your hip sockets and your spine and upper arms are more or less parallel to the floor. Try to keep your elbows from sliding away from each other (the folded nonskid mat can also help with this), and keep your head placed in neutral, with the back of the neck and skull long, the crown of the head pointed directly at the counter, and your ears right between your biceps (Figure 18A).

As you breathe here, lengthen your tailbone away from the crown of your head, and feel your pelvis lifting up and over the thighbones. Press your palms together and relax your shoulders from the inside, feeling the shoulder blades widen away from the spine and more space open in your upper back. You may also feel this stretch in the tops of the shoulders, in the triceps muscles of the upper arms, and possibly in the hamstrings as well. Allow all the stretching muscles to gently let go as you hold this pose for 30 seconds to 1 minute. Come out by walking forward, keeping your elbows supported on the table or counter, until you can easily stand all the way up.

For a deeper stretch, practice this with a block between your hands. (Figure 18B). In this version, the block keeps the both the forearms and upper arms parallel to one another, creating more space between the shoulder blades and more stretch in the muscles of the upper back, shoulders, and arms. Place the block between your hands, holding it between flat palms and pressing into the block with the roots of the fingers and the space between the thumb and index finger. Place your elbows exactly shoulder-width apart on the edge of the counter or table. Keep the fingers long and pointed upward, with the elbows bent at right angles, and practice as above, taking care not to let the elbows slide farther apart as you walk back into the stretch.

FIGURE 18B
SUPPORTED SHOULDER-STRETCH POSE, WITH BLOCK

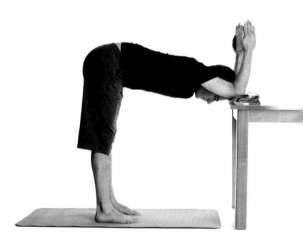

Downward-Facing Dog Pose

ADHO MUKHA SVANASANA

▼ ▼ ▼ ▼ ▼ ▼ ▼ STRETCHES THE WHOLE BODY

• RELIEVES LOWER BACK AND SHOULDER TENSION

• IMPROVES POSTURE AND GENERAL ENERGY

CAUTIONS: Practice with care in case of
hamstring, low back, wrist, or shoulder injuries.

PROP: 1 nonskid mat

OPTIONAL: 1 wedge or 2nd nonskid mat • a wall

Come onto your hands and knees
on your mat. Draw your sitting
bones back toward your heels while
stretching your arms out in front of
you, with your hands on the floor,
placed shoulder-width apart. Keeping your arms long and straight
and your hands grounded in front
of your shoulders, tuck your toes
under. On an inhalation, lift your
knees off the floor, straightening
your legs and lifting your hips up

FIGURE 19A
DOWNWARD-FACING DOG POSE

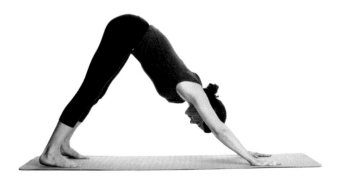

and back (Figure 19A). If the hand position is difficult for your wrists, try placing a wedge or folded mat under the heels of the hands, so the heels of the hands are higher than the fingers (Figure 19B).

Hold Downward-Facing Dog Pose for 30 seconds to 1 minute, breathing gently. Your feet should be hip-width apart and parallel with one another. Let your head rest in neutral between your arms, with your neck relaxed. Keep your hands grounded and energized. Pressing down firmly through the roots of the fingers and the inner hands—the spaces between the thumbs and index fingers—helps to open the shoulders as well as the crucial nerve pathways between the shoulders and the hands.

While breathing in the pose, lift your torso away from your hands and arms, and lengthen your spine. As you stretch upward through your sitting bones, simultaneously stretch downward through the legs, allowing your heels to move closer to the floor. Keep your legs straight, with the quadriceps muscles firm and lifted and the thighbones drawing back against the hamstrings. Gently activate the abdominal muscles, lifting into the body, so the belly feels concave and the pelvis is lifted away from the spine from underneath.

To come out, come back onto your hands and knees on an exhalation. Repeat this pose several times, if you like.

At the wall. This varia-

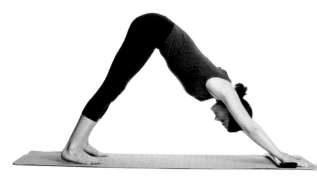

tion stretches the muscles of the hands and prevents carpal tunnel syndrome and other hand conditions related to computer and PDA use.

Place the short end of your mat against the wall. Come onto your hands and knees facing the wall, with your hands and arms shoulder-width apart. Place your hands at the wall, with your fingers turned away from each other and the inner index fingers and thumbs against the wall and the inside of the thumb pad (the muscle base of the thumb and the space between the thumb and index finger), as close to the wall as possible. As in the previous version, a wedge or a rolled mat can be used to lift the heels of the hands to lessen the angle of bend in the wrist joint, which will help reduce the pressure on sensitive wrists. Draw your hips back toward your heels, until your arms are stretched straight out in front of you, and continue with Downward-Facing Dog Pose (Figure 19C).

Please note that, as with many of these poses and exercises, this one should be practiced with caution and avoided altogether if it is painful or causes numbness. While stretching the muscles of the hands is great for prevention, it can exacerbate existing nerve conditions, especially when the damage is severe.

OPPOSITE:
FIGURE 19B
DOWNWARD-FACING DOG POSE, WITH FOLDED MAT

RIGHT:
FIGURE 19C
DOWNWARD-FACING DOG POSE, AT WALL

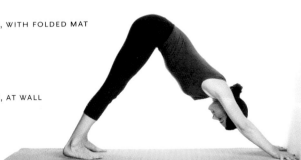

Gentle Sleeping Yogi Pose

SUKHA YOGANIDRASANA

▼ ▼ ▼ ▼ ▼ ▼ ▼ STRETCHES THE HIP AND LOWER BACK MUSCLES •
RELIEVES LOWER BACK TENSION

CAUTION: Do not practice this exercise after the seventeenth week of pregnancy.

PROP: 1 nonskid mat

OPTIONAL: 1 blanket • 2 straps

Lie on your back on your mat, using a blanket to give the spine more cushion-ing if necessary. Bring both knees up toward your chest, and reach between your legs to take hold of your feet. Holding onto either the arches or the heels (whichever is more comfortable) and keeping the knees bent and the ankles flexed, bring the feet up, so the soles of the feet are facing the ceiling and the heels are directly above the knees. The knees stay bent at approximately 90 degrees, with the calves perpendicular to the floor (Figure 20A).

If you are tight in the hips and lower back, it may be difficult to keep hold of the feet and still find correct alignment in the pose. In that case, you can loop straps around the feet to extend your reach, holding the ends of the straps, so the shoulders and neck can stay relaxed (Figure 20B). Another option is to sim-ply take hold of the backs of the thighs, around the hamstrings. The important thing is to get the legs into position, not how high you can reach.

With the legs still bent at 90-degree angles and the heels directly above the knees, relax in the hip sockets, and begin to bring the knees closer to the floor on either side of your rib cage. The knees will not touch the floor, so do not strain or use force. As the knees come lower, keep the top of the sacrum and the lower lumbar spine (the small of the back) pressing into the floor. The lower the knees come, the more you can focus on releasing the back in the other direction, thinking of uncurling and lengthening the tailbone and working more of your sacrum back to the floor.

Relax and breathe in the pose for 30 seconds to 1 minute. To come out, let go of your feet and bring your knees into your chest. You can hold there for a few more moments, allowing the thighbones to relax toward the belly and the low back to round. Then roll to one side before sitting up.

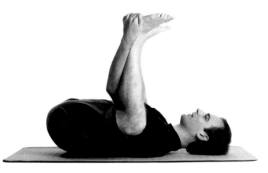

ABOVE:

FIGURE 20A
GENTLE SLEEPING YOGI POSE

RIGHT:

FIGURE 20B
GENTLE SLEEPING YOGI POSE, WITH STRAPS

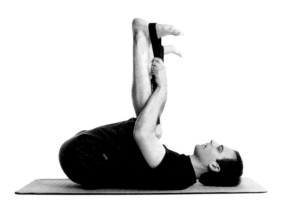

Reclining Twist Pose

JATHARA PARIVARTANASANA

▼ ▼ ▼ ▼ ▼ ▼ RELEASES THE SPINE, SHOULDERS, AND OUTER HIPS
• RELAXES THE BACK MUSCLES • INCREASES SPINAL MOBILITY

CAUTIONS: Practice with care in case of shoulder, spine, or sacroiliac injuries.

PROPS: 1 nonskid mat

OPTIONAL: 1 or 2 blankets

Lie down on your back on your mat, with a blanket spread under you for more padding, if desired. Draw both knees up toward your chest, with your thighbones dropping in toward your belly. Open your arms, and let them rest out at your sides in T position, palms facing up.

FIGURE 21A
RECLINING TWIST POSE

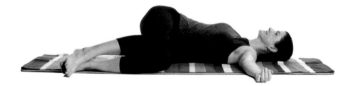

On an exhalation, begin to roll to the right, letting both knees drop toward the floor, left on top of right, as you come onto your right side. Keep your left arm stretched out to the left, but don't force the shoulder to stay on the floor. If it feels awkward, shift your hips slightly toward the left arm as you come farther onto your right side. Keep your head in neutral, with the back of your head resting on the floor and your nose pointed directly toward the ceiling (Figure 21A). Relax and breathe, feeling the back muscles loosen their grip on your spine, as the legs and the left arm drop away from each other, on opposite sides, toward the floor. Keep the left shoulder and arm very relaxed, which will help open the chest and create healthy traction for the upper spine.

If this exercise feels intense for your back at first, you can modify it by placing a folded blanket to the side you are moving toward, so your legs can rest on the blanket and don't have to drop all the way to the floor (Figure 21B).

Hold this stretch for 30 seconds to 1 minute. To come out, let the legs draw you again onto your back, leading with the top leg and letting the bottom leg follow. Then repeat to the other side.

FIGURE 21B
RECLINING TWIST POSE, WITH BLANKET

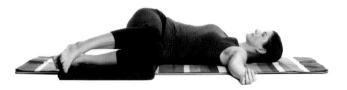

Bound Angle Pose

BADDHA KONASANA

▼ ▼ ▼ ▼ ▼ ▼ RELEASES THE HIP AND LOWER BACK MUSCLES •
INCREASES MOBILITY IN THE HIP SOCKETS FOR HEALTHY POSTURE

CAUTIONS: Practice with care in case of hip or groin injuries.

PROPS: 1 nonskid mat • 2 blankets • a wall

OPTIONAL: 2 blocks • a timer

This pose is a great antidote to a day of sitting in a chair, car, or airplane. It can be practiced toward the end of your yoga session or on its own, for a short break or transition time.

Set a timer to help you keep track of your hold time and also to allow you to relax more fully, knowing that the timer will signal you when it's time to open your eyes.

Start by placing your mat at a wall. Spread one blanket on top of your mat and fold the second blanket into thirds to create a firm pillow. Place this folded blanket at the end of your mat, against the wall.

Sit on the second blanket with your back against the wall, and fold your legs so the soles of your feet are pressed gently against each other and your knees drop out to the sides. Scoot back, so the base of your spine is firmly supported on the wall, and bring your feet close to you, with the heels close to the folded blanket, letting the outer edges of the feet rest on the spread blanket, lower than your hips (Figure 22A).

If it is comfortable, allow your legs to simply drop toward the floor, relaxing into gravity (but never pushing your knees toward the floor). If this position creates too much stretching sensation in the inner groins or outer hips, place a block under each knee (Figure 22B). Alternatively, if no blocks are available, you could try crossing your ankles instead of placing your feet against one another. This will also reduce the stretch on the muscles that hold the thigh-bones in their hip sockets. Look for a position in which you can let the legs relax completely.

Once your legs, hips, and back are all comfortable and adequately supported, rest your hands on your knees, palms face up, allowing your shoulders to relax and your arms to drop easily. Let your chin drop just slightly toward your chest,

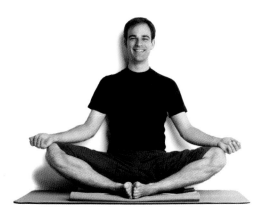

FIGURE 22A
BOUND ANGLE POSE

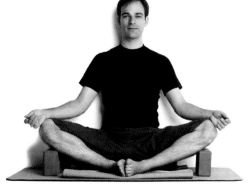

FIGURE 22B
BOUND ANGLE POSE, WITH BLOCKS

and relax your throat and the root of your tongue. Close your eyes and let your whole face soften, particularly the muscles between the jawbones and between the eyebrows. Bring your attention inward and onto your breath. Feel yourself relaxing more deeply and your awareness dropping deeper inside with each exhalation. If you find your mind racing, you can use Breathing Awareness (see page 68) to help you create a quieter energy and let go of your thoughts. This is a time to rest your brain as well as your body.

Hold this pose for 2 to 10 minutes, working up to the longer time as the pose becomes more comfortable with practice. To come out, place your hands under your knees to help lift them toward each other, and bring your feet flat to the floor before moving off your blanket.

Letting Go Pose

SAVASANA

▼ ▼ ▼ ▼ ▼ ▼ ▼ DEEPLY RELAXES BOTH MIND
AND BODY • SUPPORTS NATURAL RECUPERATIVE ABILITIES
AND OPTIMUM HEALTH

CAUTION: Do not practice this pose past the seventeenth week
of pregnancy. Lie on your side instead.

PROPS: 1 nonskid mat • a timer

OPTIONAL: 2 blankets • 1 bolster • 1 blanket • 1 eye pillow or 1 washcloth

Lay out your mat, and spread a blanket on top of it for extra padding, if desired.
The second blanket can be folded to create a small pillow for the head and
neck; it should support the cervical spine (the vertebra of the neck) but not
elevate it. Setting a timer for the length of time you want to stay in relaxation
will help you to move fully into the pose, freeing you from any worry about
how long it has been, when to come out, or falling asleep.

Lie down on your back and take a few moments to get as comfortable as
possible. Placing a bolster or a rolled-up blanket under the backs of the knees
can help create more ease in the lower back, and an eye pillow or folded washcloth over the eyes can encourage a deeper relaxation. Using these options will
enhance your experience of Letting Go Pose.

Once you are comfortable, close your eyes and begin to let go. Let your arms rest at your sides, with the palms turned up and the backs of your hands resting easily on the floor. Allow your knees and your feet to relax gently away from one another (Figure 23). Let your belly feel soft and open, and experience the rise and fall of your breath from the inside, feeling yourself surrender completely into relaxation, dropping more fully into the pull of gravity and the support of the floor with each exhalation. Let each inhalation be a reminder to clear your mind and let go of any thoughts.

FIGURE 23
LETTING GO POSE

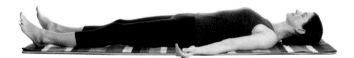

Hold this pose for a minimum of 5 minutes. Although there is no maximum, 10 to 15 minutes is ideal. When the timer goes off, stay relaxed and continue to focus fully on your breath for a few more moments, rather than jumping up. Experience what it is like to consciously and fully relax. For most of us, this is a learned skill and not a natural instinct. Ours is a culture of doing rather than relaxing, and many people find Letting Go Pose challenging at first. Although this pose can be practiced on its own any time you need a break, often it is easier for the nervous system to let go and relax into the parasympathetic (rest and restore) mode following yoga practice than it is to simply lie down and clear your mind in the midst of a busy day. In fact, you can think of your asana practice as a kind of warm-up for this pose. Following the work and sensation of the stretching exercises, your body, nervous system, and mind are more prepared for the art and deep healing of relaxation. With more yoga experience, the nervous system becomes trained, and this pose becomes more accessible. Eventually it will become easy to simply move into a deeply relaxed, meditative state without as much physical preparation.

To come out, move gently and with awareness. On an inhalation, bend your knees and place your feet flat on the floor or bolster. With the following exhalation, turn onto one side and rest there for a few more moments, so both your spine and your mind can transition slowly back into the world. The eye pillow will slip off by itself, but keep your eyes closed and let them adjust to the light coming through your eyelids before you open them. Finally, when you are ready, use the support of your arms to push yourself back up to a sitting position, looking down at the floor on the way up, so your head is the last thing to come up. Try to bring the mindful and relaxed spirit of Letting Go Pose with you as you move back into the active world.

Part Four

Putting the Poses Together

▼　▼　▼　▼　▼　▼　▼　▼　▼　▼　▼

Yoga Practice Guidelines

KEEP THE FOLLOWING suggestions in mind to get the most out of your practice.

Make a note. I find it extremely helpful to make a note of my intended practice time on my daily calendar and also to include it on my to-do list for the day. I recommend using either or both of these methods to help ensure that your yoga practice doesn't get crowded out of your mind or your schedule, as both tend to fill up with other tasks in the course of a busy day.

Space. It is wonderful to have a dedicated space for practice, if you can manage it. I've always dreamed of a house with its own yoga room, but so far, living in a one-bedroom apartment, my practice space is also my living room and my office. Clearing some furniture out of the way and setting up my home yoga studio each morning is the start of my practice, and I try to make a conscious ritual out of this process, to mark a clear physical and energetic boundary around my yoga practice.

Many of the exercises recommended in this book can be done sitting your chair in front of your computer. For a more involved yoga session, the only physical requirement for your practice space is enough room to spread out your mat and move around on it a bit; some privacy and quiet are bonuses. Most of the poses in this book can be done in a small space without much, if any, modification. Whether you have a whole room, a large closet, or a corner of your office available, and whether or not you have to set up and dismantle your personal yoga studio each time you practice, it is always helpful to set up an appealing space for yourself.

Turn off any fluorescent or overhead lights; if there is no natural light in your space, light a candle or two, placing them where you won't knock them over as you move through your asana sequence. Set your computer to sleep mode and, if it has a distracting screen saver or blinks when new e-mails arrive, drape a cloth over it. Unfurl your mat and place any props you will be using within easy reach. Arrange for a comfortable temperature (by opening or closing windows or using a fan or a space heater); yoga developed in a tropical climate for a reason, and it is not advisable to stretch your muscles when your body is cold. Do what you can to ensure some quiet, uninterrupted time. Turn off your cell phone and, if possible, the ringers of any other phones in or around your practice space. If it is noisy in the vicinity, some pleasant music playing at a low volume may help cut down on distractions. Request that your family, roommates, or coworkers not disturb you for the duration of your practice. A locked door can create extra privacy.

While it is not necessary to do all of this for a five-minute stretching break at your desk (and it is important to regularly take those short, efficient yoga breaks during your computer sessions, in addition to treating yourself to longer practice times!), taking just some of the above steps will help make even an in-office yoga break more enjoyable and effective. Creating an environment that supports your practice will help you give yourself over to it, and the benefits of a focused practice are greater than when your practice is scattered and distracted. However, if you are practicing in the midst of your workday or family life, realize and accept that not every practice session will be perfectly tranquil. And if you are under deadline pressure or having a busy, demanding day, it is better to do what you can for self-care without breaking stride (and thus creating more stress for yourself), rather than waiting for perfect conditions and abundant time to present themselves. If we required these, most of us would rarely, if ever, practice at all! We can aim for perfection, but part of developing a successful, consistent practice is accepting that we can't control all the variables and learning to tune inward, regardless of what is happening externally.

Timing. Likewise, it is ideal to practice early in the morning before eating, but more important than practicing at the perfect time or the same time every day is finding ways to fit practice into your daily life on a regular basis. On your lunch hour (before eating!) or late-afternoon coffee break, at the end of your workday, or in the evening after the kids are in bed can all be good practice times, depending on which exercises you are doing. A more vigorous practice is better earlier in the day, while the more relaxing exercises can help you wind down, as you transition from work to evening activities or prepare for sleep. Many people find that a gentle yoga session, with some easy stretching and relaxation, is more effective than a nap for re-energizing.

Eating. It is best to practice with an empty stomach, and most yoga guidelines advise not eating for two to three hours before practicing. With today's busy schedules, this isn't always possible! If you are hungry, you will not be able to practice effectively, so if fuel is needed, eat lightly; fruit, yogurt, or some kind of healthy shake or smoothie are all good choices. If you want to practice when your stomach is full, choose stretches that don't require you to compress the abdomen or invert the torso. Many of the seated stretches may be perfectly comfortable, but avoid twisting, forward-bending, and upside-down positions. In other words, it is possible to find ways of practicing even if timing and conditions aren't ideal. Regular, frequent practice is the foremost goal.

Clothes. Loose, comfortable clothes that are easy to move in are best for yoga practice. These include dance wear, T-shirts and leggings, and sweats or shorts with an elastic waist. Those of us who work at home often wear sweats and the like throughout the day, but if you are at an office and can't change your clothes, there are still some things you can do to be more comfortable for practice. These include taking off your shoes and jacket, loosening or removing belts and ties, undoing any buttons or zippers that are overly constricting. Unless you need them for safety, take off your glasses as well, since your focus is meant to be directed inward.

You want to be able to move as freely and comfortably as possible as you do yoga. For just a 5- to 10-minute stretching break, you will probably make only the minimum clothing adjustments needed to make your movements comfortable (and eliminate any risk of damaging your work clothing). Most of the at-the-computer exercises, for example, can be done without removing your shoes. But for any longer practice sessions, adjust for maximum comfort and freedom of movement whenever possible. Yoga is traditionally practiced barefoot, and removing your shoes will free up both your movement and your energy. Since we both stand and lie down on our yoga mats, be aware of hygiene issues when practicing with shoes on; you can designate one side of your mat to be used for shoes and the other for longer, barefoot practice and for lying down, or use two separate mats.

Props. The following props are used for the exercises outlined in this yoga program. I suggest starting with a minimum amount of equipment—a chair and a yoga mat are essential—and adding more as needed. You will discover through experience what additional props will support and enhance your practice. In the meantime, it is often easy to substitute with items that are usually on hand; see the suggestions that follow. Information about purchasing yoga equipment can be found in Resources.

Mat. A nonskid mat is essential for yoga practice. These days, yoga mats come in many different types. When you are choosing, keep in mind that the traction a mat provides, to prevent you from sliding around on the floor, is more important than cushioning.

Chair. A stable chair is required: this means no wheels or other moving parts! A metal folding chair without arms, of the type found at any large office supply store, is ideal. If one of these is not available, a basic wooden chair can work for most of the exercises. Make sure that your chair is placed in a stable position where it won't tip over or slide out from under you when you are using it. The best chair for yoga is quite different from the chair typically used at workstations. For sitting at your computer, a flexible, adjustable chair with wheels, arms, and a back for support is a better ergonomic choice. So you will need to have a separate yoga chair on hand.

Blanket. Blankets for yoga should be firm, because they will be folded up and used like pillows for extra support or height as often as they are used for cushioning. Eventually you will probably want to have at least two blankets suitable for yoga practice.

Wedge. Foam wedges are a recent and extremely useful innovation in yoga equipment. Because they help reduce the angle of extension and the amount of weight on the wrists in positions that bear weight on the hands and arms, they are essential for those with wrist conditions. But they perform a variety of other functions as well, and they can be useful when placed under the sitting bones to adjust posture in seated positions. If you don't have a wedge on hand, a yoga mat folded several times can often be used instead.

Strap. Yoga supply companies sell belts and straps made specifically for yoga, but for many of the exercises here, a bathrobe sash, an old necktie, or even a hand towel can substitute. Most often the strap is used to extend your reach, so whatever you use should be at least 3 to 4 feet long.

Block. Yoga blocks have many uses. They are generally used for support or to raise the level of the floor so you don't have to reach down farther than your flexibility allows. Many types are available, including traditional wooden blocks, lightweight foam, and eco-friendly recycled cork. Until you know which size and type you want, you might try using large, heavy books, such as dictionaries, which can substitute for blocks in many cases.

Eye pillow. An eye pillow is an inexpensive luxury and a useful tool for deepening relaxation and increasing the stress-reducing benefits of relaxation poses. When used for Letting Go Pose, eye pillows produce a physiological response that encourages the body and mind to drop more deeply into a relaxed state. While most people find using an eye pillow enjoyable, some do not like the sensation of having the eyes covered. So, while eye pillows are worth trying, they are not for everyone. They should only be used if they enhance, rather than detract from, your experience of relaxation. Although the weight of an eye pillow on the forehead is pleasant and has particular benefits to the nervous system, a simple folded washcloth or hand towel placed over the eyes can substitute to some extent. These will at least help shut out the light and cut down on the temptation to open your eyes and look around.

Timer. A timer is an extremely useful practice tool, especially for allowing you to close your eyes and relax fully without worrying about falling asleep and missing your afternoon meeting! A simple kitchen timer will work. The digital types are best because they are silent until they go off.

As you learn your way in your yoga practice, you may find other items useful. Experiment to find the right height for the exercises that require the support of a table or desk (a kitchen counter is a good height for many people), and make use of what is on hand, such as pillows and towels, to optimize your practice.

If you find you prefer having your knees elevated in Letting Go Pose, you may want to treat yourself to a yoga bolster. Although a firm rolled blanket or a couple of pillows will perform this function, a bolster, available from yoga supply companies, provides a bit more support and can enhance your experience of the pose. Relaxation is an essential component of yoga practice, with deep healing benefits, so use any props you like (eye pillow, bolster, blankets) to facilitate the most restful, enjoyable, and thus beneficial completion of each practice session.

Cautions and Working with Injuries

The program outlined in this book focuses on preventing injuries, not treating them. A medical condition requires care from a qualified medical professional.

It is important to note that some of these exercises, while helpful for maintaining a healthy musculoskeletal system and preventing the onset of RSI and other problems, may exacerbate an existing condition.

For each of the exercises, you will see some cautions to be aware of, including the words "practice with care" in cases of certain injuries. While yoga can often be helpful for rehabilitation, dealing with injuries in the context of a book is tricky. It is impossible to cover every possible contingency or address every potential physical condition. Although we give general guidelines in yoga, seldom do we say, "No one with condition X should do this pose." How particular movements affect different bodies is highly individual; some people with RSI benefit from stretching, while others find that it worsens their pain. Likewise, some carpal tunnel sufferers find it beneficial to do weight-bearing poses on their arms, and some find it unbearable. Downward-Facing Dog Pose is a wonderful pose for some people with diagnosed disk disease, while others with the same condition find that it puts too much stress on their damaged vertebral joints. Yoga is a multifaceted physical discipline, one that can have deep therapeutic benefits (both healing and preventive) when practiced appropriately, but it is not a medical treatment unless used with direct, qualified supervision.

In my experience, it most effective to experiment and to listen to what your body tells you about what makes it feel better and what is best avoided. The one thing we know for sure is that the human body does better when it gets lots of movement and exercise, and it suffers when it doesn't. That said, I am a firm believer in avoiding pain, and I advise *never* to push through a movement or sensation that feels risky or dubious. It is always preferable to err on the side of caution, to be patient and mindful, and to gradually increase your physical capacities, including range of motion. We all have an inherent wisdom that knows the difference between healthy sensation and actual pain, and we need to tune in to and respect what our bodies tell us, rather than going with what we wish they would say! So the intention of the words "practice with care" is to support you in doing just that and in using your yoga practice to discover and respect your own body's needs and limits.

Optimizing Benefits

Vary your practice. The concept of countermovement is a key component of RSI prevention, so the more variety you can give your body as you move through your day, the more effective your self-care program will be. This means that, although you never want to push or overstrain when you are stretching or practicing yoga, resist the temptation to do only the most enjoyable stretches. In order to change the patterns in our bodies, we have to work on movements and exercises that don't come naturally. If you do an especially hated exercise often enough, gently but consistently, you will often find that it becomes a natural and even welcome part of your routine. This is true even of relaxation, which is the most challenging aspect of yoga practice for many people. Try to bring an attitude of exploration and persistence to your whole practice, confronting the most challenging foe with an open mind and playful spirit.

More is more. The more you practice yoga, in terms of both frequency and duration, the greater the results. Yoga is neither a quick fix nor a one-time cure, but adding it to your life will ensure that you keep reaping its benefits. As you begin to use this book, start looking for how and when you might carve out practice time, both mentally and practically. We have already discussed the physical requirements for a yoga practice space, but you will probably find yourself facing other challenges as you begin your self-care program. These might include finding or making time to slow down in a busy schedule, which means making your own well-being a priority. These issues often are not resolved easily. Working with them is a process.

Practice wisely. Your practice is meant to relieve your symptoms and should never make them worse. While a certain amount of sensation is to be expected when beginning to stretch overly tight or underused muscles, and the sensation can sometimes be intense, especially at first, it should not actually be painful. Yoga should be practiced with care and awareness, looking for a sense of ease and working within your own limits. Avoid straining or pushing, and under no circumstances ever practice to the point of pain or numbness. Our bodies have great internal wisdom, and, with just a little experience, we can easily learn to recognize the difference between healthy sensation and actual pain, which is always a signal that something is wrong and that you should ease up on or avoid the activity altogether. Your practice should always leave you feeling better, and practicing regularly and gently for just a short time will teach your nervous system to welcome the sensation that comes with these stretching exercises.

Practice with joy. In addition to practicing the exercises that challenge you, which are often the ones that create the most profound change over time, also be sure to do those exercises that feel great and that you look forward to. Learning to practice yoga can be a great pleasure, as you explore and expand both your physical limitations and your kinesthetic intelligence. Yoga practice should both create change and feel good. A balanced practice is a joyful one.

Yoga Practice Sequences

Here are several suggested series of poses of varying length and focus that you can use to guide your practice. It is best to vary the sequences, depending on the amount of time you have and what your body feels like it needs at the time. If you gradually work up to doing each one a couple of times a week, you will feel enormous benefit.

MAKING SPACE

Take regular stretching breaks of 5 or 10 minutes throughout the day!

Each of the poses in the Desktop Yoga section, or any combination of them, can be used for a short break from work. It can be hard to tear yourself away from a project in progress or take time out when you are facing a deadline, but the results—a healthier body, a clearer mind, and more contented spirit— are always worth it. See if you can stretch at regular intervals—say, every 2 hours—and work your way through these poses once or even twice over the course of the workday.

TAKE A BREAK

15 Minutes at Your Desk

- Seated Posture, Figure 1A or Figure 1B
- Seated Mountain Pose with Basic Arm Stretch, Figure 2A or Figure 2B
- Reverse Prayer Pose, Figure 3A or Figure 3B

- Seated Back Bend Pose, Figure 6A or Figure 6B
- Chair Dog Pose, Figure 13
- Seated Twist Pose, Figure 7
- Seated Forward Bend Pose, Figure 10

WORKING YOGI

30 Minutes at the Computer

- Seated Posture, Figure 1A
  or Figure 1B
- Seated Mountain Pose with
  Basic Arm Stretch, Figure 2A
  or Figure 2B
- Reverse Prayer Pose, Figure 3A
  or Figure 3B
- Seated Eagle Pose, Figure 4A
  or Figure 4B or Figure 4C
- Seated Cow Pose, Figure 5A
  or Figure 5B
- Chair Dog Pose, Figure 13
- Seated Back Bend Pose, Figure 6A
  or Figure 6B
- Seated Twist Pose, Figure 7
- Seated Thread-the-Needle, Figure
  8A or Figure 8B
- Chair Standing Forward Bend
  Pose, Figure 9
- Seated Forward Bend Pose,
  Figure 10
- Seated Neck Stretches, Figure
  11A to Figure 11E
- Seated Lion Pose, Figure 12
- Breathing Awareness and
  Meditation, Figure 15A
  or Figure 15B
- Inverted Legs Relaxation Pose,
  Figure 14A or Figure 14B

ENERGIZING PRACTICE

30 Minutes for Morning or Evening

- Standing Side Stretch Pose,
  Figure 18
- Supported Spine Stretch Pose,
  Figure 17
- Supported Shoulder Stretch Pose,
  Figure 18A or Figure 18B
- Downward-Facing Dog Pose,
  Figure 19A or Figure 19B or
  Figure 19C
- Seated Eagle Pose, Figure 4A
  or Figure 4 or Figure 4C
- Reverse Prayer Pose, Figure 3A
  or Figure 3B
- Seated Back Bend Pose, Figure 6A
  or Figure 6B
- Seated Twist Pose, Figure 7
- Seated Thread-the-Needle, Figure
  8A or Figure 8B, and/or Seated
  Forward Bend Pose, Figure 10
- Seated Neck Stretches, Figure
  11A to Figure 11E
- Seated Lion Pose, Figure 12
- Breathing Awareness and
  Meditation, Figure 15A
  or Figure 15B
- Inverted Legs Relaxation Pose,
  Figure 14A or Figure 14B
- Letting Go Pose, Figure 23

EVENING TRANSITION

20 to 30 Minutes to Unwind and Relax

- Standing Side Stretch, Figure 16
- Downward-Facing Dog Pose, Figure 19A or Figure 19B or Figure 19C
- Seated Eagle Pose, Figure 4A or Figure 4B or Figure 4C
- Seated Neck Stretches, Figure 11A to Figure 11E
- Seated Lion Pose, Figure 12
- Seated Twist Pose, Figure 7
- Seated Thread-the-Needle, Figure 8A or Figure 8B
- Standing Forward Bend Pose, Figure 9

- Seated Forward Bend Pose, Figure 10
- Reclining Twist Pose, Figure 21A or Figure 21B
- Gentle Sleeping Yogi Pose, Figure 20A or Figure 20B
- Bound Angle Pose, Figure 22A or Figure 22B
- Inverted Legs Relaxation Pose, Figure 14A or Figure 14B
- Letting Go Pose, Figure 23

Part Five

Everyday Yoga

▼   ▼   ▼   ▼   ▼   ▼   ▼   ▼   ▼   ▼   ▼

ULTIMATELY YOGA IS not just an exercise program but a tool for expanding consciousness through mindfulness. So bringing yoga practice into your daily life will greatly increase the benefits it can bring. Below are some ideas for how mindfulness in your daily activities can further support RSI prevention and healthy back maintenance and augment your stress reduction program.

Yoga Throughout the Day

Practice being ambidextrous! As our bodies develop, almost all of us get into the unconscious habit of overusing our dominant side. Over time, the muscles on this stronger side begin to pull much harder on our skeletons, causing physical imbalances that produce aches and pains and making us more injury-prone. Begin to practice using your nondominant side in daily activities that don't require a great deal of small muscle dexterity. Stirring a pot of soup or sautéing vegetables, opening doors, and even reaching for something on a high shelf or reaching behind to scratch your back are all examples of movements that you can learn to do with the noninstinctive arm, simply by consciously reminding yourself to work against habit. In addition to strengthening your weaker side and balancing the body, teaching yourself new physical habits also strengthens the brain by breaking up mental patterns and increasing proprioception, thus improving your physical IQ. In terms of computer use, learning to switch your mouse hand can be immensely helpful, and although the first few days or weeks can feel awkward, with practice the muscle coordination of the non-dominant hand will improve significantly.

Balance your load. Wearing a backpack is better for your shoulders than carrying a heavy bag on one shoulder. If you must carry a purse, get into the habit of regularly alternating which side you wear it on. And try to lighten your load as well; don't carry more around with you than you absolutely need.

Keep moving. Don't limit your stretching to yoga practice sessions. You use your shoulders, arms, and hands all day long. Healthy range of motion requires maintaining a balance between strength and flexibility. So begin to treat your muscles to regular stretches throughout the day to keep them in good working order. Good times for extra shoulder stretches include first thing in the morning; after lifting or carrying anything moderately heavy (a suitcase, a grocery bag, a baby); following cooking, gardening, or driving; and at the end of the day before bed.

Strengthen your core. Strong abdominal muscles are a key component of a healthy back, so consider supplementing your yoga routines with some regular core strengthening work. Judith Hanson Lasater's book in the Rodmell Press Yoga Shorts series, *Yoga Abs,* is a great resource for this. In addition to doing targeted abdominal exercises, try replacing your office chair with an exercise ball. Sitting on the ball rather than a chair will keep your body more active as your muscles, particularly the core muscles that directly support your spine, continually make small adjustments to keep you balanced.

Lift carefully. Many people hurt their backs by lifting something that is too heavy, either because they don't know how to lift correctly or because they are trying to carry too much. It is important to lift using the strength of your legs, and this is not easy to do when you have to lean down to lift something heavy off the floor. If you have to lift a large object, protect your back by getting help. And if you have a choice, keep in mind the following advice, which came from one of my first yoga teachers and has stayed with me all these years: "Your legs are the strongest part of your body. Using them protects your back." In other words, don't try to carry all your grocery bags or suitcases at one time; make a couple of trips. You get more exercise that way as well.

Unplug. Time management is a pressing issue for most of us in this increasingly fast-paced world. Look for places to slow down. When possible, disconnect from your computer, PDA, and cell phone. Consolidate your e-mail time, reducing the number of times you check it each day as well as the amount of time you spend responding. Let the less urgent messages wait, and give yourself enough response time to allow for thorough, measured replies. Consider taking a day or the weekend off from your computer each week. If such a thing seems impossible to contemplate, experiment with it a few times; see what happens if you do unplug for just a day or two.

The most helpful measure I've taken is not turning on the computer at all until after my morning yoga practice. Checking e-mail first thing was a time thief that too often led to a truncated or missed practice session, and changing my routine to reflect healthier (and truer) priorities has been a boon. Of course, there are days when something truly cannot wait, and attending to it sometimes does mean less practice time that day. But try to be realistic about what actually requires immediate attention, rather than letting your computer and phone control how you spend your time.

When I first started taking Sundays off from the computer, two things surprised me: The first was how little of importance generally came in between Saturday night and Monday morning. The second was how restful and liberating it felt to unplug and how much I came enjoy my day off. I take care now to stray from this ritual only for something truly urgent, and few communications rise to this level.

Daily Mindfulness Practices for Stress Reduction and a Healthy Immune System

Practice yoga when you need it most. Begin to practice mindfulness in daily life. Bring your awareness back to your breath when you find yourself in stressful situations, such as slow traffic, deadline pressures, or boring meetings. Instead of focusing on the cause of the stress, watch your breath and your thoughts with the same sense of observation and acceptance that you bring to your yoga practice, and feel your body and blood pressure relax. With this practice you will see that, although you can't always control the source of your stress, you can affect your own reaction to it.

Make relaxation a daily habit. For your health, it is important to make time for relaxation on a regular basis—every day, if possible. Think of rest just as you might view taking your vitamins—as something that fortifies your whole system and keeps you tuned up to optimum capacity. On a busy day, when you really have only five minutes for practice, consider making Letting Go Pose the priority.

Create a balanced life. Health is about balance, and a life that is all work is out of balance. Taking care of yourself, doing the things you most enjoy, and spending quality time with the people you love should not be limited to vacations or delayed for retirement. Building time into your daily life for joy is not self-indulgent: it's essential for a healthy existence.

Resources

▼ ▼ ▼ ▼ ▼ ▼ ▼

Yoga with Sandy Blaine

Visit **www.sandyblaine.com** for information about classes and workshops.

Public classes, all levels
Alameda Yoga Station
2414-A Central Avenue
Alameda, CA 94501
(510) 523-9642
www.alamedayogastation.com

Advanced studies
and teacher training classes
The Yoga Room
2640 College Avenue
Berkeley, CA 94704
(510) 273-9273
www.yogaroomberkeley.com

Address inquiries to sandy@alamedayogastation.com. Please note that she cannot diagnose your condition, and cannot give you individual advice about RSI or other health concerns by phone or e-mail.

Ongoing public yoga classes are not geared toward rehabilitative work and cannot always be easily adapted for individual needs. If you have an acute condition such as RSI, work with a qualified teacher one-to-one to set up an individual therapeutic program, or look for workshops that address your particular condition.

Yoga Clothing and Props
Photographed in Yoga for Computer Users

Hugger Mugger Yoga Products, (800) 473-4888, www.huggermugger.com

Lululemon Athletica, (877) 263-9300, www.lululemon.com

Marie Wright Yoga Wear, (800) 217-0006, www.mariewright.com

Meco Corporation, (800) 251-7558, www.meco.net

Recommended Reading

Lasater, Judith Hanson, Ph.D., P.T. *30 Essential Yoga Poses: For Beginning Students and Their Teachers.* Berkeley, CA: Rodmell Press, 2003.

———. *Relax and Renew: Restful Yoga for Stressful Times.* Berkeley, CA: Rodmell Press, 1995.

———. *Yoga Abs: Moving from Your Core.* Berkeley, CA: Rodmell Press, 2005.

Mehta, Mira. *How to Use Yoga: A Step-by-Step Guide to the Iyengar Method of Yoga for Relaxation, Health and Well-Being.* London: Southwater, 2006.

Mehta, Silva, Mira Mehta, and Shyam Mehta. *Yoga: The Iyengar Way.* New York: Knopf, 1990.

McCall, Timothy, M.D. *Yoga as Medicine: The Yogic Prescription for Health and Healing.* New York: Bantam, 2007.

Rentz, Kristen. *Yoga Nap: Restorative Poses for Deep Relaxation.* New York: Marlowe & Company, 2005.

Sapolsky, Robert M. *Why Zebras Don't Get Ulcers: A Guide to Stress, Stress-Related Diseases, and Coping.* New York: Owl Books, 2004.

Holly Lloyd is a technical director at Pixar Animation Studios in Emeryville, CA, and the mother of two amazing girls, Alexandra and Madeleine. She started yoga in 1997, a year after fracturing a vertebra falling off a horse. Despite bouts of RSI resulting from computer work, Holly has kept up her office yoga with Sandy Blaine at Pixar and at other yoga classes around the San Francisco Bay Area.

Doug Sweetland has been an animator at Pixar Animation Studios since 1994, and currently is directing *Presto,* a short film scheduled for release in 2008. He started practicing yoga under Sandy's instruction in the late 1990s, at the onset of RSI complications. Those complications have been abated by yoga, exercise, and, thanks to his wife and son, working normal hours. Doug thanks Pixar for subsidizing yoga for its employees as well as for finding such a supportive instructor as Sandy Blaine.

About the Author

▼ ▼ ▼ ▼ ▼ ▼ ▼

Sandy Blaine has been practicing yoga since 1987 and has been teaching full time in the San Francisco Bay Area since 1993. In 1995 she graduated from the Advanced Studies Program at The Yoga Room in Berkeley, California, and she joined their faculty in 2000. She is a cofounder and codirector of the Alameda Yoga Station, where she teaches public classes. She has been the in-house yoga teacher for Pixar Animation Studios since 1994. Her writing has appeared in *Ascent*, *Yoga + Joyful Living*, and *Yoga Journal*, and she is the author of *Yoga for Healthy Knees: What You Need to Know for Pain Prevention and Rehabilitation* (Rodmell Press, 2005).

REVIEWING PHOTOS
ON THE SET: MODELS
HOLLY LLOYD AND
DOUG SWEETLAND,
STANDING;
AUTHOR SANDY BLAINE
AND COPUBLISHER
DONALD MOYER,
SITTING.

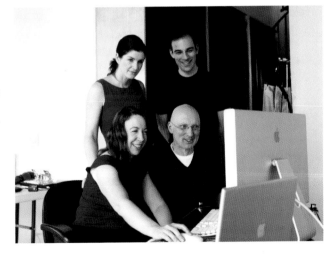

From the Publisher

▼　▼　▼　▼　▼　▼　▼

Rodmell Press publishes books on yoga, Buddhism, aikido, and Taoism. In the Bhagavadgita it is written, "Yoga is skill in action." It is our hope that our books will help individuals develop a more skillful practice—one that brings peace to their daily lives and to the earth.

We thank those whose support, encouragement, and practical advice sustain us in our efforts. In particular, we are grateful to Reb Anderson, B. K. S. Iyengar, Wendy Palmer, and Yvonne Rand for their inspiration.

Catalog Request

(510) 841-3123 or (800) 841-3123

(510) 841-3123 (fax)

info@rodmellpress.com

www.rodmellpress.com

Trade Sales/United States,

International

Publishers Group West

(800) 788-3123

(510) 528-5511 (sales fax)

info@pgw.com • www.pgw.com

Foreign Language

and Book Club Rights

Linda Cogozzo, Publisher

(510) 841-3123

linda@rodmellpress.com

www.rodmellpress.com

Index

▼ ▼ ▼ ▼ ▼ ▼ ▼